THE DEFINITIVE GUIDE TO
PROSTATE CANCER

THE DEFINITIVE GUIDE TO

PROSTATE CANCER

EVERYTHING YOU NEED
TO KNOW ABOUT CONVENTIONAL
AND INTEGRATIVE THERAPIES

Aaron E. Katz, MD

RODALE.

© 2011 by Aaron E. Katz, MD

All rights reserved. No part of this publication may be reproduced or transmitted in any form or by any means, electronic or mechanical, including photocopying, recording, or any other information storage and retrieval system, without the written permission of the publisher.

Rodale books may be purchased for business or promotional use or for special sales. For information, please write to:
Special Markets Department, Rodale, Inc., 733 Third Avenue, New York, NY 10017

Printed in the United States of America

Rodale Inc. makes every effort to use acid-free ♾, recycled paper ♲.

Book design by Chris Gaugler

Library of Congress Cataloging-in-Publication Data is on file with the publisher.

ISBN 978–1–60961–310–5

Distributed to the trade by Macmillan
2   4   6   8   10   9   7   5   3   1   hardcover

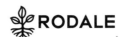

We inspire and enable people to improve their lives and the world around them.

www.rodalebooks.com

This book is dedicated to my patients. It is an honor and a privilege to be entrusted with your care.

CONTENTS

INTRODUCTION

THE GOOD NEWS ABOUT PROSTATE CANCER

One in every six men will be diagnosed with prostate cancer in his lifetime. In 2009, an estimated 192,280 new prostate cancer diagnoses were delivered. Since yearly screening with the prostate-specific antigen (PSA) blood test has become the norm for most men over the age of 50, the number of diagnoses has risen dramatically. And diagnoses of prostatic intraepithelial neoplasia, or PIN, have risen as well. PIN isn't cancer, but it's a warning sign that cancer is more likely to develop in the prostate gland. More than 30,000 men die from prostate cancer yearly. It's the second most common cause of cancer-related death in men and the second most common cause of cancer death overall.

If you are reading these words, chances are you're a recently diagnosed man or you're someone special in that man's life. And you're probably thinking, "What could be the good news in this nightmare?" It's this: Today, prostate cancer, when detected early, is almost 100 percent curable.

After the "you have prostate cancer" bomb (or the "you have precancerous cells in your prostate" bomb) is dropped, the next step is usually to meet with a urologist to discuss treatment options. Many men and their partners come to me for further advice after these discussions. They report feeling helpless and torn, having been told that their lives are in danger if they forgo immediate treatment. Often, these are men with the smallest amount of non-aggressive prostate cancer, and they have been told to undergo 9 weeks of external beam radiation or radical surgery. There is no scientific evidence that immediate treatment is called for in these low-risk situations.

If you have recently been diagnosed with prostate cancer or PIN, you may already face a mind-numbing array of treatment options, including medical treatments that carry risks of serious side effects. Today, patients often consider incorporating alternative medicine, nutrition, and supplements into the treatments prescribed by their doctors, and it can be difficult to sort the hype from the help when it comes to choosing the best of these treatments. I wrote this book to help men and their loved ones navigate these parallel worlds of mainstream medical and holistic therapies for prostate cancer.

When I was a urology resident in the early 1990s, if a patient was diagnosed with prostate cancer, we usually just took out the gland through an incision in his abdomen or perineum (the area between anus and testicles). We did the same when a man had prostate enlargement serious enough to cause symptoms. Because this type of surgery can easily sever nerves responsible for bladder control and erectile function, incontinence and impotence were common side effects. In those days, we often didn't diagnose the disease until it had spread to the bladder, colon, or bones, making for a grim prognosis. It was a lot less fun to be a urologist back then than it is now.

Back then, we thought it was better to be safe than sorry.

Because early diagnosis was much less common at the time, more aggressive treatment was usually necessary to try to contain the disease and save the man's life. When their lives were at stake, patients could stomach the risk of impotence and incontinence associated with invasive surgery and pelvic radiation treatments. And the risk was high: More than half of men who had radical prostatectomy (removal of the entire prostate) or radiation treatments ended up impotent, and half were left incontinent by their prostate cancer treatments.

Even with all of our modern tests for early detection, some men will still require aggressive treatment. But we now know that these treatments are not necessary across the board. We have tools that enable us to discern the treatment course that is (1) least likely to cause a man to lose his ability to have sex or control his urinary function and (2) most likely to allow the man to live out his normal life span with the best possible quality of life.

Active Holistic Surveillance: An Introduction

Since early detection and close tracking have become standard, men over 70 with small cancers who don't get the radiation therapy mandate may be advised to take a "watch and wait" approach. My version of this is active holistic surveillance—where we use advanced, sensitive tools to track these small cancers, enabling us (1) to stay on top of the situation and intervene if and when necessary and (2) to use herbs, diet, and other holistic interventions to promote the body's natural defenses against cancer growth and spread.

In low-risk situations, no treatment at all may be needed. Did I say "no treatment"? Yes—I did. Read it again. *Men on active holistic surveillance or other watch-and-wait programs may never require definitive treatment.* The cancer may never spread beyond the prostate or cause any symptoms at all.

And even when treatment is needed, there's no one-size-fits-all approach. All roads do not lead to the radiation center or to the surgeon's table. There's a better way to approach this thing called prostate cancer—a more balanced, thoughtful, personalized, and targeted approach.

Although the urological center I founded and continue to run at Columbia University Medical Center is called the Center for Holistic Urology, and although I talk a lot about active holistic surveillance, what we're really doing is creating this more balanced approach by integrating what works from every discipline—holistic and mainstream medical. That's why I prefer to call this work *integrative* urology instead of holistic urology. Much more will be said about the difference between integrative and holistic medicine in Chapter 3.

I juggle a lot of roles at work: practicing urologist, professor of urology, and researcher of holistic therapies. On pretty much any day I show up at work, I teach students how to perform the latest diagnostic and therapeutic procedures, perform those procedures myself, spend lots of time informing patients so that they can choose their optimum course of treatment, and help to run and write up research studies. I know firsthand that mainstream therapies are better than ever and that alternative and nutritional therapies have their place in prostate cancer treatment and prevention.

In 2009, I got to add "talk show visiting health expert" to my weekly schedule. Don Imus invited me to talk about men's health on his televised radio program. He jokes about whether or not I've brought surgical gloves and orders me to keep my hands on the table, and I have the opportunity to share what I know with his enormous audience, many of whom would not otherwise hear the information I'm delivering.

My first book, *Dr. Katz's Guide to Prostate Health*, was a general discussion of prostate health and disease. It gave equal treatment to prostate enlargement, also known as benign prostatic hypertrophy, or BPH; prostatitis, an inflammation of the prostate gland; and prostate cancer. Although that book is still relevant, I decided a new book was needed just for men who are dealing with prostate cancer or who are at high risk of the disease. (BPH and prostatitis are dealt with in this book, too, but they don't get quite as much of the spotlight as prostate cancer.) Since the publication of my first book, many developments—across the full spectrum of conventional and holistic therapies—have taken place in the world of prostate cancer. I felt it was time for an update.

Active holistic surveillance is at the heart of what we do at the Center for Holistic Urology, and it has definitely evolved since my last book. Active surveillance isn't for everyone, however, even in some men who have these small, probably slow-growing cancers. Some men may feel too much anxiety about not treating cancer, even if we know that those cancer cells—which are indeed cancer cells in the classic definition—are not likely to ever cause harm. Others may not want to follow the schedule of repeat PSA testing commonly used to check for disease progression or to follow the diet and take the nutritional supplements that I feel are so important. Fortunately for these men, we can now offer targeted, focal treatments for early-stage prostate cancer that carry much lower risks of side effects than some of the older procedures that treat the entire gland.

It's important to note here that *whether men with early-stage prostate cancer choose to go on surveillance or not, they can still benefit from the holistic treatments described in this book.* The holistic therapies described here can be of value to men with more advanced disease, too—and they are definitely good choices for men who are at high risk for developing prostate cancer and wish to take a proactive approach toward prevention.

Whether men with prostate cancer choose to go on active holistic surveillance or opt for immediate treatment, this book gives them the power to make the most informed choice for their individual case and to help themselves heal regardless of the course they choose. Holistic treatments can also be used to broadly support men with more advanced cancers who require mainstream therapies, all of which are explained in detail to help men make the best possible treatment choices. Men who undergo mainstream prostate cancer treatment can also use the Center's integrative program to reduce risk of a recurrence.

Holistic Prevention

If you have not been diagnosed with prostate cancer, perhaps you have relatives who have been diagnosed with the disease and you've discovered that this means you are much more likely to get the same diagnosis. You might be in what your doctor has called a high-risk group and you're trying to be proactive about prevention. Or you may be one of a growing number of men who've had prostate biopsies and found that you don't have cancer but you do have prostatic intraepithelial neoplasia (precancerous cells growing in your prostate gland). You're hoping that there's something you can do to stop those precancerous cells from becoming cancerous.

If you belong to one of these demographics, the program outlined in this book will suit you well—as long as you're genuinely interested in proactive prevention. It will promote your non-prostatic good health in many ways, too. Cardiovascular and immune health can be improved with the same holistic interventions I recommend for prostate disease.

What to Expect from This Book

This book explains prostate health and prostate cancer treatment to men and their loved ones in simple, straightforward language. It also gives readers tools to shift diet, exercise habits, and stress-coping techniques to patterns that help the body combat cancer while promoting mental clarity, energy, balanced good health, and longevity.

Read this book and share what you've learned with your medical team; they might learn something from it that will benefit you as you navigate this journey. Also share what you're learning with your personal support team—partners, friends, family members. As you prepare yourself to heal from or to prevent prostate cancer, you can only benefit from their encouragement and support.

PART I

LAYING THE GROUNDWORK: YOUR PROSTATE, CANCER, AND MODES OF TREATMENT

CHAPTER 1

YOUR PROSTATE: A USER'S GUIDE

Let's be honest: The relationship between a man and his reproductive system is probably the most important one in his life. And as with every relationship that matters, we tend to take it for granted.

When everything works just right, men get to enjoy some of life's greatest pleasures: attraction, sex, desire, the making of children. And when everything is working right, why try to understand how it all operates? That would take all the romance out of it.

At a certain point, however, it becomes important for a man and his reproductive system to get acquainted in a whole new way. This time comes right around midlife—the point at which things can start to go wrong "down there." For a substantial proportion of men, sexual function or libido might decline. Urinary difficulties might start to show up. Or a routine physical might lead to a diagnosis of prostate problems: enlargement of the prostate gland, a urinary tract infection, a questionable result from the blood test used to detect prostate cancer (the PSA screening test), or even prostate cancer.

Many men have never really thought about the fact that their bodies contain prostate glands until they receive a diagnosis of prostate disease. Few men know much about where this gland is or what it does until it starts to malfunction (or, as is often the case, until cancerous cells are detected long before any malfunctioning becomes evident—which can seem like an ambush to a man who feels great one moment and becomes a cancer patient the next). But a lot of men are getting this wake-up call.

In the late 1980s, urologists began to use the PSA blood test to detect prostate cancer. Since that time, diagnoses have become far more common. Overall, the rate of prostate cancer diagnosis has risen by 67 percent since the middle of the 20th century. Today, 18 percent of men can expect to get a diagnosis of prostate cancer at some point in their lives. And just under 20 percent of men ages 55 to 74 develop some clinical signs of benign prostate enlargement.

Rates of prostate cancer are rising in part because of earlier detection and in part because the population is aging—prostate cancer is primarily a disease of older men. However, because of routine screening with the PSA test, we are now detecting this cancer in men in their forties and fifties. Getting to know your prostate couldn't hurt, because chances are good that you're going to end up addressing one or another prostate issue in your lifetime.

It's Okay to Be Scared . . .

My best guess is that there's only one reason you have this book in your hands: You or someone you love has been diagnosed with prostate cancer or is at an especially high risk of developing the disease. Taking this step to inform yourself is commendable, especially if you're doing so in the days or weeks just after receiving a cancer diagnosis. This period of time can certainly be an emotional roller coaster.

If you are feeling traumatized and wish you weren't, or think that if you were truly manly, you wouldn't be feeling fearful or sad, you should know that these feelings are significant and in no way inconsequential. There's research to prove this: In one Harvard Medical School study of 350,000 men diagnosed with prostate cancer between 1979 and 2004, rates of suicide and death from heart attack and stroke—both of which can be linked to psychological stress—jumped during the first months following diagnosis.

The good news here is that this spike in death rates in the months following diagnosis stopped after 1993, when early detection efforts began in earnest. When the prognosis is good—as it is when prostate cancer is diagnosed in its earliest stages—the trauma is much less severe than when the cancer is diagnosed after it has spread too far to be curable. When the issues you face have more to do with making treatment choices in the interest of healing than with having to acknowledge a grim prognosis, psychological health isn't likely to crash and burn. You know you can do a lot to help yourself.

One reason for the enormous stress that used to accompany a prostate cancer diagnosis was the level of risk most treatments entailed—treatments that could be devastating to that all-important relationship between a man and his reproductive system. When I was a medical resident in the early 1990s, about half of men who underwent treatment for prostate cancer ended up impotent. Half ended up with urinary incontinence. The significant risks of impotence and/or incontinence made treatment choices close to impossible to make for some men.

Over the past 2 decades, death rates from prostate cancer have fallen, and treatments are now head and shoulders above what they once were, in terms of both effectiveness and reduced risk of side effects. Our rates of survival and cure from this disease are the highest ever, and in the last decade we have made many great advances in our understanding of the biology of prostate cancer cells, which has led us to vastly improved treatments.

Most important, we are learning that many men diagnosed with prostate cancer using modern early detection techniques *do not need immediate treatment.* A proportion of these men may never need treatment at all. That is why I believe this book is so needed: Men and their loved ones need to know that they can make an educated choice to postpone treatment, and they need a measured and up-to-date perspective on how to make this choice for themselves. In addition, they need to know that "watch and wait" can become a much more empowered process of "watch, wait, and act" when the holistic strategies described in this book are employed.

If you're not familiar with the idea of holistic therapies, you might imagine that they're about as valid as voodoo, astrology, alien abduction, or psychokinetics. But the reality is that herbal medicine, diet, and other "alternative" therapies are now converging with mainstream science-based, evidence-based medicine. One of the places where this is happening is my Center for Holistic Urology. In this book, I will not recommend any holistic therapy that does not have a solid basis in scientific validity and peer-reviewed research studies—for the most part, the same kinds of studies done on the drugs approved by the FDA and prescribed by doctors every day.

My primary aim in this book is to provide you with all the information you need following a diagnosis of prostate cancer, even if you are living with the disease and ongoing tests show that the cancer may have come back after treatment. To put all of this information to good use, you'll need to make a deeper, more detailed acquaintance with your prostate gland and with some other parts that reside in the same general neighborhood in the male body.

Your Prostate: An Overview

The prostate gland is actually an integral part of the reproductive system. Situated underneath the bladder, wrapped around the urethra (the tube that carries both urine and semen out of the body), and nestled up against the front side of the rectum, the prostate is a gland made up of multiple lobes and encased in a membrane. The section of the urethra that passes through the prostate is the *prostatic urethra.*

A healthy young man's prostate weighs in at just over ¾ ounce and is roughly the size of a large walnut or a small plum. During the buildup to ejaculation, the prostate secretes liquid through small pores that lie between it and the prostatic urethra. This liquid nourishes and carries sperm as they pass through the urethra on their voyage out.

On either side of the prostate sit *seminal vesicles,* which are small, pouchlike glands that contribute secretions to semen. Next to the seminal vesicles are *Cowper's glands,* which produce fluids that lubricate the urethra. Right at the confluence of these vesicles with the top of the prostate gland, two delicate *vas deferentia* (translation: vessels that carry away) also enter the urethra. Each of the vas deferentia extends from one of the testicles and up and around the bladder to get where they need to go.

The testicles, of course, are where sperm are produced. Immature sperm convene in the *epididymis* on top of each testicle. They mature there and wait for their big chance—the next ejaculation— at which point the vas deferentia contract rhythmically and draw sperm out to their date with destiny. Testicles also produce testosterone, the hormone that gives men sexual drive and the ability to have an erection. Testosterone also causes the growth of the prostate gland. One of the ways we can cause cancer to regress is to remove the ability of the testicles to produce this hormone. Today, we can do this surgically or with medications.

You may recognize the word root *vas* as the same one that initiates that dreaded word *vasectomy*—a procedure that severs or closes off these tubes to prevent sperm from leaving the body. It's interesting to note that some studies have found a link between vasectomy and prostate cancer. If you've already been through this procedure, you probably can't blame your prostate problems on it. Today, most evidence fails to support any connection between vasectomy and prostate cancer.

Prostate-specific antigen (PSA), the enzyme measured in the bloodstream by the PSA test, is produced within the prostate. Its purpose is to keep semen liquid so that it flows easily. When semen enters a woman's vagina, enzymatic reactions cause the this. And the size of a man's prostate does not necessarily predict whether he will need treatment for prostate enlargement. Some prostates grow outward without squeezing the urethra and limiting urine flow. At the other extreme, a man's prostate can grow only a small amount, but because it expands inward, it can restrict or stop the flow of urine, making treatment essential. (I'll address prostate enlargement in much more detail in Chapter 11.)

The tissues and cell type of the prostate gland are actually very similar to the tissues that make up female breasts. Breasts are made up of lobes that produce fluid and ducts that allow that fluid to pass out of the lobes and be concentrated in one place; so is the prostate gland. Both types of tissue also control the flow of the fluids they produce. Like breasts, the prostate is highly sensitive to sex hormones like estrogen and testosterone. Unlike breasts, the prostate is partially made up of muscle, which contracts during ejaculation to move prostatic fluids into the urethra and to move semen along on its path.

Although a man with prostate disease isn't likely to want to think about this point too much, the prostate gland is also a sexual organ. It is sensitive to stimulation and plays an important role in the overall sensations of orgasm. Some men have discovered this for the first time while having a digital rectal exam at the doctor's office. It's not unusual for a man to become aroused or even to ejaculate during a DRE. The prostate has even been called "the male G-spot."

Now that you have the general lay of the land, let's look at what can go wrong with this small bit of male pelvic real estate. Although the emphasis in this book is on prostate cancer, I'll start sperm to clump up in a gel-like mass at the entrance to the cer vix. Within a half hour, PSA dissolves the gel, allowing sperm t swim for their ultimate goal—to fertilize an egg and make a ne human being.

In a healthy prostate, very little PSA escapes from the gland into the bloodstream. Thus, an elevated PSA level may be a reflec tion that some pathological process is going on within the gland.

The PSA test is *not* a cancer test. A finding of elevated PSA can indicate several conditions. It may be cancer, or it may be prostatitis (a non-cancerous inflammation of the prostate), or i may be just a large prostate due to a benign growth, otherwise known as benign prostatic hyperplasia (BPH). Ejaculating or getting a digital rectal exam (DRE) will also make PSA rise You'll learn everything you ever wanted to know (and perhaps more) about PSA in Chapter 7, where this topic is addressed in great detail.

Most men's prostate glands grow bigger and heavier as they age. At birth, a baby boy's prostate weighs a little less than ½ ounce, and it goes through growth surges in adolescence and in the mid-twenties. It's normal for a man's prostate to grow again start-ing in his fifties, in part because of changes in hormone balance that are typical of men in midlife. The average man's prostate enlarges by about one-quarter in the last half of life.

Some men's prostates grow more than others. Surgeons at Weill Cornell Medical College reported removing a prostate gland that weighed *18 ounces* from one patient—it was the size of two grapefruits, big enough to fill the man's entire pelvis with prostate tissue. Enlargement is usually much less severe than here with the most common prostatic issue in men over 50: benign prostatic hyperplasia.

Benign Prostatic Hypertrophy, aka Prostate Enlargement, aka "the Growing Problem"

As I mentioned earlier, a substantial percentage of men in midlife and beyond develop BPH serious enough to cause urinary problems. They may notice that they have to get up to urinate more often during the night or that they need to urinate more in general. Difficulty starting the urine stream, weak urine stream, small urine volume, feeling of not having emptied the bladder completely, or blood in the urine can all suggest BPH. These can also be symptoms of prostate cancer, so any man I see in my office who is complaining of symptoms like these will be evaluated for both conditions.

Despite intense research over the past few years, medical science isn't sure what causes the prostate to enlarge and result in BPH. There are two predominant theories, both of which have to do with changing hormone balance during the midlife years and beyond. Neither theory has been proven conclusively, and neither theory seems to explain every case of BPH.

As a man ages, his production of the masculinizing hormone testosterone decreases. Men's bodies also produce estrogens, which are thought of as female hormones but are actually produced in the adrenal glands of men's bodies, as well as in stored fat. Estrogen is a growth promoter: It stimulates the growth of tissues—particularly those of the sexual organs, including the prostate. Thus, BPH may result when estrogen production stays the same while testosterone production diminishes.

A form of testosterone called dihydrotestosterone (DHT) is believed to play a significant role in BPH. It has a directly stimulating effect on prostate tissue—in other words, it makes prostate tissue grow. Studies have demonstrated that if no DHT is present, prostate enlargement doesn't happen (on a side note, male pattern baldness also requires the presence of DHT). Heightened DHT levels in the prostate are linked with greater risk of prostate enlargement.

Genetics can play a major role in BPH. In my practice over the years, I have found that younger men whose prostates grow very large and who have urinary symptoms are more likely to have had a close relative with this condition—usually their father. If a man knows that a close relative has had significant BPH that required treatment, he may be more likely to require something beyond holistic treatments: medications like Avodart, for example, which can reduce prostate size.

Although mild BPH isn't dangerous, it can lead to bigger problems if left untreated. Urinary tract infections can begin to develop as urine is retained in the bladder. The kidneys can be damaged if there is high pressure in the bladder that moves up into the kidneys. In rare cases, it can lead to swelling of the kidneys, which is known as hydronephrosis ("water on the kidneys").

Standard treatments for BPH include medications like 5-alpha reductase inhibitors (which decrease the amount of dihydrotestosterone in the prostate, which then shrinks the gland's tissues) or alpha-blockers (drugs that reduce muscle spasms that can contribute to constriction of the urethra in BPH). Neither drug works for everyone, and both have side effects.

For BPH, I often start out with herbal remedies like saw palmetto, pumpkin seeds, *Pygeum africanum*, and stinging nettle, especially in men with mild urinary symptoms. These herbs can spare many men the need to use pharmaceuticals. I haven't seen any side effects with these remedies. On the other hand, I don't recommend herbal compounds to men with moderate to severe symptoms, and there is *no* role for herbal therapies in men who have clear cases of urinary retention.

Behavioral modification—reducing the number of diet sodas or caffeinated drinks consumed each day, for example—can help reduce BPH symptoms.

Surgery may be the best course for some men with BPH. These surgeries have been refined a great deal since my medical school days, when we just took out the whole gland, often mangling nerves necessary for continence and potency in the process. Today, we use high-tech arthroscopic methods to surgically remove just enough of the prostate to restore good urinary tract function.

At this writing, the state of the art in surgery for BPH is the green light laser procedure. It has been a big success in terms of effectiveness and lack of side effects as a replacement for the older transurethral resection of the prostate. This minimally invasive outpatient procedure can be performed in under 20 minutes with light anesthesia. We have experienced very high patient satisfaction in response to this procedure. You'll learn more about BPH and its treatments in Chapter 11.

Prostatitis

Put simply, prostatitis is an inflammation of the prostate gland. It's the most common prostate ailment in men under the age of 50.

Prostatitis is a fairly mysterious entity. Sometimes it hurts, sometimes it doesn't; sometimes it's caused by bacteria, sometimes no infection is present to explain the inflammation. When it's bacterial, curing it is usually as simple as a course of antibiotics. But in most cases it's not bacterial, and finding relief can take some time and effort. A detailed explanation of prostatitis—symptoms, causes, and potential solutions—is offered in Chapter 12.

Prostate Cancer

The bulk of this book is about cancer of the prostate: what it is, what the risk factors are, how it might be prevented, how it's detected, how it's treated, and how to reduce the chances of recurrence. In the next chapters, you'll get a good feel for what you're up against, whether you:

- are currently being treated for or were recently diagnosed with prostate cancer, whether isolated to the prostate or spread beyond its borders

- have had a high PSA test but have not been diagnosed with prostate cancer

- have had a biopsy and received news that you have prostatic interepithelial neoplasia (the appearance of precancerous cells in the prostate) or are in a high-risk group (for example, African American men or men who have close relatives who have had prostate cancer) and want to take preventive steps—and to be prepared if and when you do face a diagnosis of prostate cancer

- have a partner, loved one, or family member who is dealing with any of the above

When it comes to treatment options, patients face much more complex choices than they did when I was in medical school in the 1990s. In some instances, cancer is detected so early that it may not require treatment—and if it's slow-growing, it may *never* require treatment. PIN is not usually treated at all but can be watched carefully with repeat testing. When prostate cancer does require treatment, options may involve more than one type of surgery (open, robotic, or cryotherapy), radiation, or hormone-blocking drugs.

Surgeries in particular have improved dramatically since the turn of the millennium; the risk of side effects has dropped a great deal. In chapters to come, I'll explain in detail each kind of procedure and its potential benefits and risks. This book gives special focus to *cryosurgery*, where cancer cells are targeted (with the help of ultrasound scanning) and literally frozen to death using tiny needles. I authored a book on this procedure and teach it worldwide to medical students, residents, and urologists. I use it often in my urological practice, and I believe it's one of the best avenues for men who require surgery. Patients who opt for cryosurgery have a low risk of side effects, recover quickly, and are out of the hospital the same day! For many men diagnosed with early-stage prostate cancer, active surveillance (rather than immediate treatment) may be a terrific choice. This type of surveillance, with possible delayed intervention, has become much more popular in recent years, now that we know many of these cancers may never cause any harm.

A growing body of research is demonstrating the effectiveness of natural medicines such as herbs and nutrients, specific dietary changes, and stress reduction in slowing prostate cancer growth and suppressing recurrence. These holistic therapies are at the heart of the chemoprevention and active surveillance programs I design and prescribe at the Center for Holistic Urology. Unlike most other books on this subject, this book offers men research-supported herbal and nutritional therapies that have shown promise in slowing the growth of prostate cancer cells and even reversing the progression of PIN. As the hazards of mainstream medical therapies become better understood by the public, and as interest increases in holistic, natural ways of combating illnesses, more men are seeking out alternative therapies for prostate disease. Men with PIN or small, slow-growing cancers can use the Center for Holistic Urology's chemoprevention program to put off surgery, drug therapy, chemotherapy, and radiation—or even avoid them altogether.

While the idea of preventing or reversing cancer with nutritional and herbal therapies and alternative medicine gets plenty of media attention these days, much of what's being promoted lacks a solid foundation in scientific research. Chemoprevention revolves around high-caliber research-based natural therapies that slow or reverse the growth of cancers.

Strategies for early detection of cancer—prostate and others—have made a big difference in our ability to cure patients. The problem with early detection is that we can detect cancers that might not necessarily require aggressive treatment. Mainstream medicine tends to treat aggressively anyhow, and this is expensive and risky when treatments involve surgery, radiation, and powerful chemotherapy and other drugs. With chemoprevention, we can take a gentler approach, sparing patients the potential side effects of more invasive treatments and sparing the health care system some major expenditures.

The information given about prostate cancer chemopreven-tion will benefit the health of every man, whether he has prostate cancer or not. Heart and bone health benefits are welcome "side effects" with this holistic approach.

Following a nutritional plan like the one described in Chapters 8 and 9 gives men the power to do much more than watch and wait; it gives them tools they can use to heal themselves proactively. Holistic treatments can also be used to support men with more advanced cancers that require mainstream therapies, all of which are explained in detail to help men make the best possible treat-ment choices. Men who undergo mainstream prostate cancer treat-ment can use the Center's integrative program to reduce the risk of a recurrence. This book will allow many more men to benefit from the work we've been doing at the Center for Holistic Urology.

CHAPTER 2

UNDERSTANDING PROSTATE CANCER (AND CANCER IN GENERAL)

One must not forget that recovery is brought about
not by the physician, but by the sick man himself. He
heals himself, by his own power, exactly as he walks
by means of his own power, or eats, or thinks,
breathes or sleeps.
—GEORG GRODDECK, *THE BOOK OF THE IT*, 1923

During the Nixon administration, the War on Cancer was mounted. The popular belief was that if we put our collective minds and hearts into finding a cure for cancer, we couldn't possibly fail. But 40 years later, we continue to fight a disease that is poised to become the leading cause of death in developed nations. The more we learn about cancer, the more complexities emerge, and the more we realize we have to learn.

Humanity has a long history of doing battle with the dread disease cancer. It's seen as a mysterious invader, an evil force, a thing to be feared, fought, and eradicated. In decades and centuries past, cancer seemed like a mysterious monster, but today, we have a pretty good understanding of this disease. Knowing what we know now, we can at least shine a bright light on that monster and see how it operates: why it shows up, who is at risk, and how we can best prevent and combat it.

Our understanding and successful treatment of cancer has progressed in leaps and bounds even in the last couple of decades. Early detection and high-tech treatments have conspired to make survivable cancers that once were a certain death sentence. Demystifying the cancer monster will help you to replace stress and fear with a deep understanding of what exactly this entity is, how it's likely to behave, and how you can change your life in ways that will either eradicate it or cause it to grow as slowly as possible.

Cancer is actually over 100 distinct diseases, but they all have certain elements in common. In this chapter, you'll learn the basics about the big C: what it is, why it happens to some and not to others, and our best understanding of the common denominators believed to be involved in most cancers. Since this book is about prostate cancer, I'll hone in on this particular variant of cancer and all its manifestations. Let's shine some light on this cancer monster. In seeing clearly what you are up against, you hold the best chance of being an active agent in your own healing.

Some Cancer Statistics

In the United States in 2010, 1,529,560 new cancers were diagnosed and 569,490 people died from cancer. This represents a significant decline in diagnoses and deaths from years prior. Lung cancer was the most common diagnosis in men (222,000 diagnoses), with prostate cancer coming in a close second (217,730). One in every two men and one in every three women alive today will be diagnosed with some form of cancer in their lifetimes; most of them will be over the age of 65.

One in six men will be diagnosed with prostate cancer at some point, and 1 in 34 men will die from the disease. The average age of diagnosis of prostate cancer is 69, and the risk is insignificant in men under 50—with the exception of African American men and men who have close family members who have had the disease. Two-thirds of men diagnosed with prostate cancer are over 65 years of age, and African American men have a 60 percent higher chance of being diagnosed with the disease than white men. (Interestingly, Africans living in their native countries have very low risk. So do men from China and Japan. When they move to the United States, however, their risk rises substantially.)

Certain behaviors or environmental exposures can increase cancer risk. People who smoke, who are exposed to carcinogenic chemicals (pesticides, herbicides, solvents), too much sun, or ionizing radiation (X-rays, radioactivity, radon gas), who drink more than two alcoholic beverages a day, who eat poorly and don't exercise, or who are overweight are at greater risk of certain cancers. That means that a person subject to these conditions is more likely to develop cancer than one who isn't.

Being infected with certain viruses or bacteria can increase the risk of some cancers. Human papillomavirus, for example, increases the risk of cervical cancer in women, and hepatitis increases the risk of liver cancer. A family history of cancer may increase risk (this is particularly true with prostate cancer).

This being said, many people who have no risk factors at all still end up battling cancer. In this age where health information is everywhere and all kinds of hype exists about what we can do to prevent diseases like cancer, it's easy to wonder, "What did I do wrong? Did I bring this on myself? Not enough organic vegetables, maybe, or too much stress?" The last thing you need in the face of a new diagnosis is self-blame. Let that go.

For that matter, let's consider for a moment that cancer may not actually be a monster. It isn't out to get you. It's just a collection of cells whose genetic coding has gone awry, and it almost always does so for a reason. In understanding those reasons, you don't have to take responsibility for having caused it, because—as you'll see—not all of the risk factors for this disease are under your control. But you can use a lot of this information to move toward a cancer-free future.

Cancer: A Very Brief Introduction

The human body is made up of about 50 trillion cells. A lung cell, a skin cell, a breast cell, a stomach cell, and a prostate cell are all different from one another and do specialized work in the body. In their DNA, they carry genetic "programming" that tells them how to develop and behave, how quickly to reproduce, and when to die.

Cell death might not sound like a good thing, but a cell that knows when it's time to kick the bucket provides space for a new, healthy cell to take its place. This process is essential for the health of tissues and organs. In cancer medicine, this healthy kind of death is called apoptosis. Much of the research into drugs and natural therapies for cancer begins with studies of cancer cells in test tubes, where we add the substances being studied to those cell cultures to see whether apoptosis is enhanced. More apoptosis is a good thing—it indicates a slowing effect on cancer's growth.

A group of healthy cells (also known as a cell line) given the right amount of nourishment and growth medium will continue to renew itself—old cells dying and new cells forming to take their place—for a predictable period of time, at which point the entire cell line dies. This amount of time is known in medical research as the Hayflick limit.

Cancer cells have no Hayflick limit. They can be kept alive and thriving indefinitely. Cancer cells reproduce abundantly; they have no "off switch." Certain alterations in cells' DNA cause cells to become immortal: They stop dying when they're supposed to die.

A single small sample of tumor tissue can be kept alive and grown to make more samples, which can then end up being used in cancer research laboratories all over the world. A cell line taken in the 1950s from the cervical tumor of Henrietta Lacks, a thirty-one-year-old African American woman, has been used in over 60,000 cancer research studies. In a single laboratory—the lab of Columbia researcher Vincent Racaniello, PhD—these so-called HeLa cells derived from Henrietta Lacks's cervical tumor have been propagated for almost 3 decades, producing some 800 billion cancer cells.

The initial transformation of a healthy cell into a cancerous cell due to changes in DNA is known as initiation. The next phase, promotion, is where some influence stimulates the growth and multiplication of cancerous cells. As these cells accumulate, they begin to become less *differentiated*, which means they become less able to do their special jobs in the body. A prostate cancer cell, for example, is good at growing and multiplying, but not so good at doing the work a prostate cell is supposed to do.

The shift from initiation to promotion can take years, even decades, and a tumor's growth can be so slow even after it has begun to accelerate that the cancer will never be a threat. (Some cancers, like leukemia, do not form tumors but affect circulating blood cells.) This is especially true with prostate cancer. In autopsy studies of men who have died from other causes, about 30 percent of men in their fifties and 60 to 70 percent of men in their eighties had small prostate cancers.

Cancers are named for the organ or type of cell in which they start. If a tumor is benign, it can grow to a large size, but it won't spread through the body. A benign tumor is not life-threatening. If a tumor is malignant, it may at some point in its growth start to spread. It can go beyond the organ in which it is growing, or tumor cells can pinch off and travel through the bloodstream or lymph system to distant places in the body. If these cells lodge somewhere and begin to grow a new tumor, this is known as metastasis. Those new tumors are still identifiable as cells from the original tumor. If lung cancer metastasizes to the brain, for example, we would call it not brain cancer but metastasized lung cancer. The word *cancer* is derived from *karkinos,* the Greek word for "crab," which is an image that accurately describes the appearance of a spreading tumor.

Risk Factors for Prostate Cancer

A risk factor is an indication that you might have a behavior, a genetic trait, or some other characteristic that has been found to be more common in people who have a particular disease. These risk factors tend to show up more often in people with that disease than without it.

In some risk factors, we have a pretty solid idea that there is an element of causality: that something about the behavior or characteristic creates a biological mechanism that then triggers the onset of the health condition. In others, we don't really know why the relationship exists, so we're not sure how to reduce the impact of the risk factor on the chances that the disease will develop. Knowledge of some risk factors can help guide us to behaviors that may help reduce risk; not much can be done about others.

A few general risk factors not under our control:

• Being male

• Being over the age of 50

• Having a family history of prostate cancer

• Being African American

• Living in the United States (an American man's chance of developing prostate cancer is much higher than the rate in many other nations)

And one risk factor we may have more control over:

• Eating a diet high in fat from meats and dairy products

In recent years, we've found that aggressive, deadly prostate cancer and slow-growing, non-aggressive prostate cancers seem almost to be two different diseases with different risk factors and ways of progressing. For example, while smoking and diets low in vegetables don't seem to be linked with slower-growing prostate cancers, they are linked to aggressive ones. Obesity is linked to a higher risk of aggressive disease, but not to the slower-growing varieties.

Fortunately, we have tools in urological oncology for distinguishing one type from the other. Although we do sometimes overtreat a non-aggressive cancer—subjecting a man to difficult treatment ordeals and potentially devastating side effects when watchful waiting and chemoprevention would have worked just fine—this is becoming less common and will become even less so as we continue to refine diagnoses and treatment plans and improve on our watch-and-wait strategies. Modern procedures like cryosurgery help us treat most prostate cancers with much lower risk of side effects like impotence and incontinence, so the question of whether or not to treat becomes easier to answer with confidence.

Cancer's Common Denominators

Beyond specific risk factors for cancers, we can ask deeper questions: What causes cancers to form? What makes them grow and spread? It's in understanding the ultimate answers to these questions that we find our way toward a cure—or, better yet, a prevention—that really works. As you learn about these common denominators, you'll see that they also help to explain the risk factors previously listed.

Although we are only beginning to answer these questions thoroughly, we do understand a few key influences that may be at the root of most cancers. Understanding these factors hasn't brought us to a cure, but they are useful in the quest to prevent the initiation of cancer and to slow its progression. Nearly all the dietary changes and nutritional supplements I'll recommend in Chapters 8 and 9 of this book are designed to help modulate these root factors in the initiation and progression of prostate cancer.

Free radicals/oxidation

Inside most cells are tiny energy "factories" called mitochondria. Mitochondria are only 5 to 10 micrometers in diameter—that's about a thousandth of the width of the tip of a pencil.

Inside these mitochondria, carbohydrate, protein, and fat molecules are transformed into energy through a complex series of biochemical reactions collectively known as respiration. Respiration creates a sort of "exhaust" called free radicals. Free radicals can do damage in many ways, including modifying cellular DNA in ways that create cancerous cells.

Chemical carcinogens (including tobacco smoke), excess exposure to sunshine or other forms of radiation, and the chronic inflammation that can result from bacterial or viral infections all increase the production and activity of free radicals, which are also known as reactive oxygen species (ROS). Runaway stress—the kind characteristic of the "type A" personality—also has the end effect of increasing levels of ROS. Nearly all these factors have been linked to cancer initiation and progression.

Add to this the fact that diets richest in foods that contain abundant antioxidants—vegetables, fruits, whole grains—have been found to be potent cancer preventives, and you'll see why so much effort has gone into researching the relationship between cancer and free radicals. If free radicals were fires, antioxidants would be water. The body also produces its own antioxidants;

exercise enhances levels of these *endogenous* (created in the body) antioxidant substances. These antioxidant substances are nature's antidote to excess ROS.

Humans are designed to strike a reasonable balance of free radical production and antioxidant intake. Given modern-day, antioxidant-depleted diets and lack of activity, plus exposure to lots of toxic chemicals, it's easy to see how that balance becomes skewed.

The chemopreventive plan offered later in this book is built partially on a foundation of enhancing natural sources of antioxidants and bringing in highly concentrated sources through herbal supplements. Exercise and stress reduction both aid in reducing *oxidative stress* (the term used to describe free radical overload).

Inflammation

When you bump your knee, twist your ankle, or develop an infection, your immune system kicks into gear to heal the injury or illness. In the process, it creates something called inflammation. Redness, swelling, heat, and pain are all created by immune cells coalescing and doing their healing work: In the case of injury, it clears out dead and dying cells and facilitates healing; and in the case of infection, specialized immune cells attack and eliminate unwanted invaders. Ideally, this kind of *acute* inflammation sets in, does its work, and then dissipates. In some cases, inflammation gets too intense, and the fire meant to cleanse and heal burns down the whole figurative house. Tissues might be destroyed or a fever might turn out to be deadly. This rarely happens in modern times, where medications for controlling infection and inflammation are readily available and often prescribed.

Sometimes inflammation becomes chronic. This can be the

case with *Helicobacter pylori,* a chronic bacterial infection of the stomach linked to ulcers; infections of the bowel that cause inflammatory bowel diseases like colitis; hepatitis infections of the liver; or infection of a woman's cervix by papilloma viruses. In all these types of infection, cancer risk is increased, and this is believed to be due to the effects of long-term, slow-burning inflammation on cellular DNA. Inflammation is a process that produces free radicals. Chronic inflammation means increased oxidative stress, which—as you learned in the previous section— also enhances the risk that healthy cells could turn cancerous.

Long-term inflammation can lead to *dysplasia,* a precursor to cancer: Cells start to exhibit abnormalities that aren't yet cancer but are likely to move in that direction. In this book, you'll learn a lot about prostatic intraepithelial neoplasia, a form of dysplasia that can be detected in prostate biopsies. It's estimated that 15 percent of cancers worldwide are attributable to chronic inflammation from microbial infections.

Behaviors and exposures linked to cancer often have an inflammatory effect on the body. For example, cigarette smoking causes chronic inflammation in the lungs, as does exposure to asbestos or silica, both of which are lung carcinogens. The same goes for throat and mouth cancers—smoking causes inflammation in the throat and mouth as well. Overexposure to sunshine or radiation causes inflammation, which helps explain the link between these risk factors and the cancers connected to them. Obesity creates a state of chronic inflammation in the body, which is one reason it may increase cancer risk.

When researchers look closely at breast tissues that have become cancerous, signs of inflammation can be seen. This is also true of prostate tissue (remember that these two types of tissue are similar) and of other cancers as well. Anti-inflammatory drugs like aspirin, ibuprofen, and naproxen—known collectively as non-steroidal anti-inflammatory drugs, or NSAIDs—are modern medicine's go-to measure for getting rid of chronic inflammation and reducing out-of-control acute inflammation. Because of what we know about the relationship between inflammation and cancer development, NSAIDs have been studied as preventive measures in people at high risk of some cancers. The most compelling results have come back from studies of people at high risk of a hereditary form of colon cancer. The subjects in these studies tend to develop precancerous polyps in their colons, and NSAIDs drastically reduce their risk of developing colon cancer.

What about prostate cancer prevention with NSAIDs? The evidence in favor of protection with these drugs isn't as clear, but it does exist. In one survey of about 9,000 men in Saskatchewan, Canada, men who had used NSAIDs were at slightly lower risk of prostate cancer than men who had not. A review of 91 studies found that daily intake of NSAIDs for 5 or more years reduced risk of colon cancer by 63 percent, lung cancer by 36 percent, esophageal cancer by 73 percent, stomach cancer by 62 percent, and prostate cancer by 39 percent. Other studies demonstrate that NSAIDs may also help slow cancer progression and metastasis.

Why, then, don't we routinely recommend ongoing NSAIDs for cancer prevention? They have some side effects that make widespread use too risky. Using NSAIDs for extended periods can erode the lining of the stomach, causing bleeding ulcers that in some cases end up being life-threatening. With some NSAIDs, risk of heart problems increases enough that ongoing use means robbing

Peter (heart health) to pay Paul (cancer prevention). The risks versus the benefits don't merit broad recommendations to take daily NSAIDS for cancer prevention—no matter how much fun that would be for the pharmaceutical companies that manufacture these drugs.

Here's the good news in all of this: *The biological mechanism believed to confer most of the protective effects demonstrated with NSAIDs can be produced in other ways.* Herbs, nutritional supplements, and dietary and lifestyle changes can have just as powerful an anti-inflammatory effect as NSAIDs, without risk of side effects. In Chapters 8 to 10, where I go into depth about chemoprevention, you will learn potentially life-extending ways to use nutrition and lifestyle shifts to either prevent or slow the development of cancer (prostate and others) while *improving* gastrointestinal and heart health. All of this is backed up by scientific research, some of which has been done in my own lab at Columbia University.

Hormone imbalances

Prostate cancer has a hormonal component. Testosterone and estrogen enhance the growth of existing cancers, and sometimes we cut off the flow of those hormones with surgery or medication to try to slow prostate cancer if we cannot eradicate it. On the other hand, men with low testosterone levels are at higher risk of prostate cancer, and the use of testosterone replacement therapy to raise their levels of this hormone does not appear to increase prostate cancer risk. Some research suggests that high levels of testosterone are protective against aggressive prostate cancer but not against less aggressive forms of the disease. Surveys of men with prostate cancer show a strong relationship between high levels of estrone, a form of estrogen, and prostate cancer risk. Obesity increases estrogen levels—and this might help explain why men who are heavy have a higher risk of aggressive prostate cancer.

The picture of hormonal effects on prostate cancer—in both the risk of developing it and the ways in which we try to slow it down once it has developed—is (to put it mildly) complex. In Chapter 6, you'll learn in detail about hormone ablation and its role in treating more advanced prostate cancer. And in the chapters on chemoprevention, you'll learn how the diet and lifestyle plan laid out in this book can help keep hormone levels in better balance, no matter what your diagnosis.

CHAPTER 3

UNDERSTANDING INTEGRATIVE MEDICINE AND ITS SCIENTIFIC FOUNDATIONS

Make no mistake: The advances and developments in biomolecular medicine that we enjoy in this country are nothing short of stunning and profound—and we must continue to pursue them with great vigor, focus, and intention. In the same way, we must continue and even further expand our explorations of the value and benefits of alternative and complementary therapies.

—JEREMY GEFFEN, MD, FACP, INTEGRATIVE ONCOLOGIST, TESTIFYING BEFORE THE CONGRESSIONAL COMMITTEE ON GOVERNMENT REFORM ON CANCER CARE FOR THE NEW MILLENNIUM, JUNE 2000

Early in my career, I was as skeptical as most of my colleagues about alternative therapies. My understanding of plants as medicines didn't go much further than what I'd been taught about illegal drugs in medical school, aside from the few medicinally valuable botanicals that had been discovered—most notably digitalis for the heart, derived from the foxglove plant.

According to the wisdom doled out to us during our expensive education as doctors, alternative therapies weren't backed by enough evidence to merit our consideration. There was no doubt in my mind that the tools of modern medicine represented the true state of the art, and I wasn't about to lead my patients, who were trusting me to heal them, down any garden path lined with medicinal herbs and meditation cushions. When I had surgeries, medications, and radiation therapies at my disposal, and when the effectiveness and safety of those tools kept improving by leaps and bounds, I couldn't see any good reason to prescribe untested, unproven dietary changes, herbal therapies, or mind/body practices like massage or visualization. All of that changed when I had a chance to work with urological patients at the Atkins Center for Complementary Medicine in Manhattan.

Between 1993 and 1997, I spent time one day each week working with urological patients at this center, which was then run by the same Dr. Robert Atkins who created the world-famous Atkins diet. (He died in 2003.) Every patient who came to the Atkins Center was prescribed nutrient supplements, dietary changes, and other alternative therapies.

Initially, my skepticism kept a strong hold on me as I observed. But I heard so many positive stories from Atkins Center patients about how alternative medicine had helped them that I had to reconsider. The evidence in favor of these alternative therapies was compelling enough to persuade me to investigate the current science on nutritional supplements, herbs, and other forms of alternative medicine.

By 1998, I was convinced that alternative approaches could be valuable for urological diseases, especially when combined with mainstream therapies. More important, it was clear to me that high-quality research was badly needed to determine which alternative medical approaches were of greatest value. That's when the Center for Holistic Urology (CHU) at Columbia University Medical Center, a research and treatment center, became a reality.

If I had tried to open a holistic urology center a decade earlier, I would probably have caused some raised eyebrows in the medical community. But with the general growth in interest in alternative medicine over the past couple of decades, the number of people who seek these therapies is rising, and the area itself is becoming increasingly well-validated by medical science.

Since the Center first opened its doors, the support of the urological medical community and its patients has been strong. Other urologists who don't use alternative therapies are glad to have a colleague to whom they can send patients who wish to include such therapies in their treatment.

You Say Integrative, I Say Complementary: Defining Medical Schools of Thought

By this point, I've referred to alternative, integrative, mainstream, and holistic medicine. What do these words really mean, and how are they involved in the advice you'll get in this book? To ensure that we're all on the same page when I use these terms, let's take a moment to define each one.

Mainstream (Allopathic) Medicine

Modern, mainstream Western medicine is *allopathic*. Allopathy is a Greek word built from two root words that mean "other than" and "disease." The term was originally coined by the 19th-century physician Samuel Hahnemann.

Allopathic medicine treats an illness with an agent or a therapy that works *against* or *opposite to* a disease process. When we treat high blood pressure with a drug that causes blood pressure to drop, that's an allopathic treatment. The same goes for antibiotic treatment of an infection, use of an alpha-blocker like Flomax to treat urinary symptoms and decrease pressure on the urethra, or radiation therapy to shrink a tumor.

In the strictest definition of the word, allopathy can refer to herbs and other natural remedies used against a disease. If we administer anti-inflammatory herbs to decrease inflammation, for example, that's allopathy. But the term *allopathic* is generally used in connection with mainstream, modern Western medicine to set it apart from alternative medicine. That's how I use it in this book.

Dr. Hahnemann was the creator of *homeopathy,* a word whose roots translate to "same as" and "disease." Homeopathy treats like with like, using minute amounts of substances derived from foods, herbs, minerals, or animals that stimulate the body's natural defenses and healing responses. Homeopathy is extremely safe, but many physicians are skeptical that it has any effect. Others, like me, have seen it work well and consistently enough to recommend it in some cases. In Chapter 9, I'll go into more depth about this issue to help you decide whether you would like to try homeopathy.

Alternative Medicine

As its name suggests, alternative medicine is an alternative to mainstream Western allopathic medicine. It can include the following therapies:

acupressure

acupuncture

biofeedback

bodywork, including massage, healing touch, or energy work

botanical (herbal) medicine

changes in diet

detoxification

exercise

homeopathy

meditation

nutritional supplements

prayer

psychological/spiritual counseling, including support groups

visual art therapy, music therapy, or other art therapy

visualization

yoga

The ancient medical systems of India (ayurveda) and China (traditional Chinese medicine) are considered alternative medicine in the United States. Both incorporate herbs, nutritional medicine, bodywork, exercise, and spiritual aspects.

About 40 percent of Americans use some form of alternative therapy on a regular basis. Exercise, diet changes, nutritional supplements, acupuncture, yoga, counseling, meditation, and herbal medicine are all finding their way into mainstream medical practices.

Holistic Medicine

The word *holistic* comes from the Greek word *holos,* which means "whole" or "in its entirety." When something is holistic, it emphasizes the relationships between its parts and the whole.

A doctor with a holistic mind-set does not walk into the examining room with the intention of isolating the patient's disease and zapping it with a magic bullet. The holistic doctor treats the whole patient, taking into account his emotional and psychological health, his life circumstances, his relationships, and the workings of his entire body (even the parts that are working just fine).

Holistic medical treatment also takes into account the importance of the relationship between the patient and his caregivers. When a doctor treats a patient as though he is less than a whole human being—just a chart, a disease, or a set of procedures—the patient may lose confidence, sensing that this caregiver is not in tune with what's really going on with his patients. This can have an important impact on the patient's ability to heal. A holistically minded doctor makes sure to listen to the patient's concerns and answer every question. He takes time to explain anything that needs to be explained and does his best to make the patient feel cared for and supported. He comes across as warm and openhearted when communicating his thoughts and feelings to the patient.

Complementary/Integrative Medicine (CIM)

To keep things simple, I'm going to use these two terms—complementary and integrative—interchangeably. They describe the same thing: a combination of allopathic and alternative medical treatments. This is what we practice at the Center for Holistic

Urology. Whether a treatment is allopathic, homeopathic, or alternative, as long as research and experience show it to be safe and effective, we will integrate it into our treatment protocols.

Although CIM is finding its way into many mainstream medical disciplines, cancer medicine (oncology) is one of its most exciting applications.

"The Terrain Is Everything"

Louis Pasteur (1822–1895) was instrumental in proving that microorganisms were a causative factor in many diseases. He clashed with another scientist of that time, Claude Bernard (1813–1878), who believed there was more to sickness than the presence or absence of certain germs. It's said that on his deathbed, Pasteur said, "Bernard was right. The microbe is nothing. The terrain is everything."

This could well be an urban myth, but its message is true. A body in a good state of well-nourished health will resist a microorganism's invasion better than a body that's not as well cared for. Genetics and other factors over which we have no control can also make that physical terrain more vulnerable to attack—but if we do all we can to keep the body in the best health possible, we have a better chance of fighting off that bug.

The same is true of cancer. While we know a lot about chemicals, genes, and germs that can trigger carcinogenesis (the development of cancer), cancer growth, and cancer spread (metastasis), many environmental factors play into the disease as well. Even in a person whose genes are geared to create higher cancer risk, external factors like diet and lifestyle impact the expression of those genes—and, by association, the risk that a cancer will form, grow, and spread. Alternative medicine can support the terrain of the body, making it less hospitable to cancer's growth.

As you already know from reading Chapter 2, cancer is a complex disease that can arise in many forms. It has the capacity to morph and change in ways that defy efforts to target and eradicate it. Early detection changes the balance of power somewhat, but the fact is that cancer can't be treated in the same way as a lung infection, a kidney stone, or appendicitis, all of which can almost always be dealt with in "magic bullet" fashion. Cancer requires that we address every aspect of the patient's physical and psychological health. With the integrative approach, we help the patient create a state that resembles—as closely as possible—balance, peace, and good health; at the same time, we use modern medical tools to try to eradicate the disease.

A healthy human body fed a nutrient-dense, sugar-free, reduced-fat diet without any red meat can do more of the work of stopping the disease in its tracks. Learning practices that reduce psychological stress changes the internal environment of the body in ways that promote a stronger healing response. Alternative therapies help the body respond better to drugs and herbs.

Even if this integrative approach doesn't eradicate all of the cancer, it will greatly enhance the patient's quality of life and probably his or her longevity. Many of the approaches that we discuss in this book are also excellent for maintaining a healthy heart and improving the vascular system (the blood vessels throughout the body). With integrative medicine, quality of life and overall health will improve almost immediately. This is why cancer care centers today are increasingly getting on board with integrative programs. The M.D. Anderson Cancer Center at the University of Texas, the Cancer Treatment Centers of America (a group of six hospitals devoted to complementary/integrative cancer care), the Integrative Medicine Service at Memorial Sloan-Kettering Cancer Center in New York City, Simms/Mann UCLA Center for Integrative Oncology, Duke University's integrative oncology program, and many others are using CIM and are participating in research that continues to close the gap between alternative medicine and Western allopathic medicine.

Proactive Patients Are Leading the Way

When Richard Nixon declared the War on Cancer in the 1970s, modern Western medical science took a characteristically militaristic approach to finding a cure: Figure out what's invading the body's terrain, then determine which drugs, surgeries, and other treatments could most accurately annihilate it. And although this approach has yielded important advances in cancer diagnosis and treatment, we can't yet roll out the victory banner. (Reminder: We're doing a lot better with prostate cancer than with some other cancers. When the disease is detected early, we can cure almost every case. In urology, we have also done very well with testicular cancer, where again the cure rates reach 100 percent. Lance Armstrong, who had testicular cancer with metastases to the brain and lungs, received intensive chemotherapy and went on to win the Tour de France multiple times following his treatment!)

Early diagnosis and high-tech treatments have gotten us to a point where survival rates are far better than they once were, but over 500,000 people still die yearly from cancer in the United

States. (That's about one-fifth of total deaths in a year.) Because cancer is not always curable by mainstream medical means—and because some mainstream cancer treatments may cause harmful side effects—patients often do research on their own to create complementary/integrative programs. In many instances, this is done without the knowledge or consent of the treating oncologist; hopefully, as integrative oncology programs become the norm rather than the exception, patients won't feel the need to hide their alternative practices from their medical teams. The use of CIM is greater in cancer patients with more advanced disease or in those who have relapsed following conventional therapies.

According to the National Health Interview Survey (NHIS), which is performed every few years by the government, just over 60 percent of cancer survivors report having used some form of alternative medicine in the past year. Most of the respondents used prayer and spiritual practices. Relaxation techniques were used by 42 percent of respondents; about 40 percent used nutritional supplements or vitamins; 15 percent reported doing some form of meditation. Massage, yoga, hypnosis, support groups, and biofeedback were also incorporated by some of these cancer patients.

It's interesting to note that male respondents in the NHIS survey were fine with diet changes and nutritional supplements but didn't much care to hit the yoga studio or the massage table. Keep this in mind if you feel yourself crossing something off your alternative therapies list because it doesn't feel manly enough. You might be cheating yourself out of something that could aid your healing.

Here's an example. Many men think of yoga as something for people who are flexible and look good in tight spandex workout gear, not for the average guy who hasn't touched his own toes since he was a toddler and whose only workout until now has consisted of shooting hoops once a week with buddies, then spending the next day on the couch sipping a cold one while nursing several pulled muscles. But yoga is actually for anyone who wants to improve flexibility, endurance, balance, and strength—really, it's best for people who think it's not for them at all!

I recently added yoga to my weekly workout routine. I chose Bikram yoga, which is performed in a room where the temperature is over 100 degrees. We do work up a very manly sweat. Stretching and straining in a saunalike room makes increasing flexibility much easier. Yoga improves circulation and reduces symptoms of arthritis, and I've found that it increases my energy levels a great deal. There are many forms of yoga to choose from, and they can all be helpful to the prostate cancer patient. You'll never really see how until you take the plunge. To find out more, refer to Chapter 10 on the roles of stress reduction and exercise in prostate cancer chemoprevention.

Which alternative methods, then, are best for men with prostate cancer or those at high risk for the disease? This question will be answered in depth in coming chapters of this book (as will your questions about mainstream treatments). You're going to learn all you need to know about allopathic and alternative treatments for prostate cancer and other prostate diseases. To support my recommendations to you, I'm going to refer from time to time to the scientific research that is at the foundation of my belief in those treatments. I'd like you to go into the remainder of this book with a basic understanding of the ways in which this research is conducted.

In Search of Evidence-Based Alternative Approaches

We live in an age where medical research moves along at a rapid pace and where treatment protocols change every day. The field of herbal research is especially exciting; never before have we been able to understand the molecular mechanisms of so many herbal compounds and their role in the management of cancer patients. While this constant evolution of treatment protocols makes it an exciting time to be practicing medicine and doing research, this same variability can make things confusing for patients.

The answer here is for patients to learn basic information about how we conduct medical research. Understanding the research process will help you understand the reasoning behind the treatment protocols we use at the Center for Holistic Urology—and it will allow you to continue to make better treatment choices as new options become available.

Almost any treatment prescribed by physicians has gone through a long, costly process of testing. The purpose of these tests—which are standard with any new compound, natural or synthetic—is to answer the following questions:

1. Is it effective?

This doesn't require much explanation. Either the treatment helps the person get better or it doesn't. Even if it isn't harmful, using any treatment that doesn't work is a waste of time and money and may take the place of a treatment that could really help.

Once scientists figure out that a substance might make a good medicine, they usually do test-tube studies on cells or organs from animals. These are called *in vitro* studies. Such studies can be done with herbs and nutritional supplements as easily as they can be done with drugs. At the Center for Holistic Urology, for example, we've done many studies in which herbs are introduced into a petri dish where prostate cancer cells are growing. We study the results carefully: Does the herb seem to slow the progression of the cancer's growth? Does it stimulate apoptosis (spontaneous cancer cell death)? What effect does it have on enzymes that regulate inflammation, which we now know to be an important factor in carcinogenesis and cancer progression? Can these herbs affect the DNA of cancer cells in ways that make them inactive and unable to cause metastases (growths of cancer distant from the original cancer site)? From answers to questions like these, we can determine which substances merit the next step, where we introduce the experimental herb or drug into the diet of research animals. These *in vivo* ("in the living body") studies can mirror what happens in the human body. They help us determine the herb's or drug's effectiveness while confirming that the compound isn't toxic.

Eventually, studies on human beings with the disease in question are needed to see whether the substance actually works as a treatment or a cure. This is where things get a lot more costly and complicated—and this is why studies on drugs, which are usually funded by drug companies, tend to get done more often and on a larger scale than studies on herbs or nutritional supplements. To do studies on human beings, subjects with the disease have to be recruited into a type of study called a clinical trial. The study group is usually divided into smaller groups, which get different treatments. At the end of the treatment period, the outcomes of the groups can be compared to discern whether any of the treatments has been effective. In urological research, we can draw our conclusions using measures like PSA (for example, what treatments made PSA go down the most?), urinary symptoms (if we're researching treatments for prostate enlargement), biopsy results, or quality-of-life issues.

Most such studies include a placebo group, which gets a sham, fake treatment such as a sugar pill. If the treatment being tested does not outperform the placebo, we can be fairly certain that it isn't effective.

The most interesting part of this—and a powerful argument in favor of including alternative therapies in treatment plans for any disease—is the fact that placebos can actually be just as effective as medical treatments. This is the power of the mind at work, and in a complementary approach, we can harness this power to promote healing. More on this in chapters to come.

2. Is it safe?

Evidence-based treatments can and do cause side effects that can be harmful. That's why, when you see a drug ad on TV, you always hear a long list of unpleasant side effects being rattled off in a pleasant voice by the announcer. They're par for the course with pharmaceuticals—if it's powerful enough to work as a drug, it's powerful enough to cause side effects.

To prove safety, researchers conduct a series of tests on animals where they look carefully for toxicity or other ill effects. If those tests go well, they move on to testing the treatment in humans—still monitoring closely and making note of any side effects that might make the treatment unacceptably dangerous.

When the end result of the clinical trial has demonstrated that the drug's or herb's benefits outweigh any risks, the investigational treatment may then become what we call the standard of care. At that point, we integrate it into protocols we use to treat patients.

Herbs and supplements are vastly safer than drugs. They are natural substances that are more easily processed by the human body. A drug is a chemical that has been built or altered from its natural state to give it more powerful or targeted effects, so it has greater potential to cause collateral damage. The number of deaths or serious injuries from supplements and herbs is minuscule compared with those that occur with prescription and over-the-counter medications.

Still, it's important to keep in mind that herbs and supplements are not always safe, especially in combination with certain mainstream therapies. If you don't have access to an integrative medical team and need to design your own integrative program with your allopathic doctors, be sure to do your homework whenever you consider adding a new herb or supplement. A pharmacist can help ensure that your proposed addition doesn't interact with your current medications and supplements.

Sometimes, high-tech surgeries, drugs, and other treatments are exactly what's needed. When a disease is aggressive or advanced, I'm not going to just have the patient sit around meditating or swallowing herbal supplements instead of having the treatments I know could be lifesaving. I'm grateful to have state-of-the-art medical tools, medications, and procedures at my disposal. I'm also grateful that oncology in general is integrating alternative medical methods.

3. Is it effective consistently enough to be recommended to most people who have a health condition?

In 2002, a book called *Living Proof* was published. Its author, British tutorial fellow Michael Gearin-Tosh, was diagnosed with a bone marrow cancer called multiple myeloma in 1994. He chose to fight the disease with alternative approaches and to reject conventional chemotherapy. He was given a year to live and ended up living for 10 years, dying in 2005 at the age of 65. Gearin-Tosh also used the Gerson therapy, along with some other more controversial natural therapies for cancer. He also used nutritional changes, herbs, and vitamin supplements.

There are many other books out there like Gearin-Tosh's. If you are telling others about your diagnosis, you're probably hearing lots of similarly inspiring tales—maybe some about people who have rejected mainstream treatments and survived cancers that had threatened their lives. Some of these true-life tales may contain valuable information. Still, *any testimonial like this is about a single person's experience.* It can't be generalized to other people with cancer. There's no telling what really helped a single person to heal. To gauge the true value of any medical treatment, you need to test it on as many people as possible.

The larger the study group, the more reliable the study's results. If I test an herb on only 10 men, I'm more likely to get an ambiguous result—one that makes the treatment appear effective when it isn't or that makes it appear ineffective when it isn't—than if I test it on 100 or 1,000 men. If we test a treatment on 10 men and 7 have a good result, the result is much less compelling than if it has a good effect on 70 out of 100 or 700 out of 1,000 men. With these higher numbers, we can safely figure that the treatment is going to work for most people who get it.

Drug studies routinely involve hundreds or thousands of people. In herbal research, however, it's difficult to get adequate funding to do studies on more than a handful of human subjects. This goes a long way toward explaining why herbal medicines haven't become standard treatments in mainstream medicine.

Follow the Money

In this book, I offer all of the research support I can so that you can make educated choices in your own holistic urological protocol, but you should know up front that there isn't as much research on these topics as my allopathic medical mind would like there to be. With the research efforts of integrative oncology centers, this is beginning to shift. Studies are getting done, although they don't match the size and scale of pharmaceutical company–sponsored studies. It's virtually impossible to get funding to do alternative medicine studies on large numbers of human subjects.

The cost of studies that demonstrate the safety and effectiveness of new drugs and lead to FDA approval can easily escalate into the millions of dollars. More study subjects means higher cost. Most of the time, bills for research studies on a new drug or medical device are footed by the manufacturer of that drug or device—the corporation that stands to profit if the treatment turns out to be a success. Supplement companies sponsor research studies on their own products, but their pockets aren't as deep as those of the pharmaceutical conglomerates or the medical device manufacturers.

With the high cost of research required for FDA approval, drugmakers need to be able to charge high prices for their products without fear of competition from other drugmakers. They achieve this by patenting their products. A product that's natural cannot be patented. Any other company can make a product just like it and sell it under a different name. Drug company patents give exclusive rights to a particular drug formulation for 7 or more years, which gives them time to recoup their investment. At that point, other companies can copy the formula and call it something else, or generic versions of the same drug can enter the marketplace at a much lower price. The way things are today, researching supplements just isn't a worthwhile investment for drug companies.

The practices engaged in by "Big Pharma" to sell enough drugs to recoup their investments can be questionable, to say the least. Big Pharma's deep pockets are the main source of financing for medical research, medical meetings, and doctors' continuing education, and drug companies rarely hesitate to put all their marketing muscle into influencing medical practice in ways that will be most profitable to them. Any marketing guru will tell you that the way to influence an industry is through a direct relationship with the individuals who are part of it. And Big Pharma does some of the best marketing on the planet. No purveyor of natural substances has the financial resources or people power to match what they do.

Doctors are offered free samples, perks, trips, dinners, trinkets, concert tickets, and honoraria in exchange for their time, allegiance, or simple presence in a place where they can be plied with the drugmaker's best marketing tactics. Imagine being offered an all-expenses-paid trip to Hawaii, a lavish dinner at a fine restaurant, or a generous honorarium just for showing up somewhere to hear a drug company pitch. Hard to resist—and although most doctors who take advantage of these perks would say that they aren't influenced by them, the reality is that the very possibility of that influence creates an unacceptable level of potential bias. More and more doctors and legislators are "just saying no" to gifts, perks, and other marketing manipulations on behalf of drug companies, but this is only a recent trend at this writing. You should know that conflicts of interest can and do influence the way doctors treat their patients in the United States, and they create a bias toward pharmaceuticals and pricey medical procedures and away from herbs, supplements, and other holistic options.

Medical research is what we rely upon to create standards for medical practice, and these conflicts of interest create a falsely positive idea of what certain medicines or procedures can do for our health. Pharmaceutical companies also fund most of the continuing medical education programs doctors must attend to keep their licensure current. I hope that this helps you begin to see where the strong bias toward allopathic treatments and against alternative treatments comes from. All you have to do is follow the money. Allopathic treatments get so much more research support because they have a lot more funding behind them.

Although guidelines designed to prevent conflicts of interest in medical research have improved in recent years—for example, in certain kinds of studies, researchers have to reveal whether they are on the payroll of a pharmaceutical company or even if they hold the company's stock—there's a lot more work to do on this front. Here's an example from the world of cardiology (the branch of medicine that diagnoses and treats heart disease). A type of study called a meta-analysis is often used to create practice guidelines in medicine. Meta-analyses gather together multiple studies on the same treatment, and all the data that went into those studies are combined to help determine whether that treatment is safe and effective. While the clinical trials that are combined in meta-analyses have to reveal all the authors' ties to drug companies, those ties do not have to be revealed in meta-analyses. In March 2011, a report published in the medical journal *Archives of Internal Medicine* revealed that more than half of almost 500 writers and reviewers who helped to create the current guidelines for treatment of heart disease were, at some level, earning money from drug companies.

In addition, industry-funded drug studies that fail to demonstrate clear benefit to drugs that have been heavily invested in by their manufacturers are far less likely to end up being published in medical journals than those that make the drug look good. This means that the body of research that goes into creating these meta-analyses—which, again, are the resources doctors use to establish guidelines for which drugs and procedures to use on their patients—tends to be biased in favor of drugs and procedures that may not be as effective or safe as they are chalked up to be.

Conversely, although much excellent research has been performed on natural therapies, many sources of information on alternative approaches are full of myth and misinformation. Studies are frequently published, but their quality is often subpar compared with that of allopathic medical research. For now, keep in mind that if some new supplement or alternative therapy hits the press and it sounds too good to be true, it probably is.

I hope that this short introduction to the science behind new treatments will be helpful to you as you move through this book and in general as you distinguish hype from help in your own investigations of alternative treatments.

PART II

WHEN THE NEWS ISN'T GREAT: PROSTATE CANCER DIAGNOSIS AND TREATMENT

CHAPTER 4

THE TRUTH ABOUT PROSTATE CANCER SCREENING AND DIAGNOSIS: WHAT TESTS ARE REALLY NEEDED AND WHY

Two decades into the PSA era of prostate screening, the overall value of early detection in reducing the morbidity and mortality from prostate cancer remains unclear. . . . While early detection may reduce the likelihood of dying from prostate cancer, that benefit must be weighed against serious risks associated with subsequent treatment, particularly the risk of therapy for cancers that would not have caused ill effects had they been left undetected.

—Andrew M. Wolf, MD, Associate Professor of Medicine, University of Virginia Health System, Charlottesville, Virginia

What you ultimately end up with here is the risk of overtreatment versus the risks of dying from prostate cancer . . . and I think most men would rather not die.

—Herbert Lepor, MD, Professor of Urology, NYU School of Medicine, New York City, New York

We need a better test than the PSA. PSA is a lousy
test. It misses as many cancers as it finds. . . . The
benefits of prostate cancer screening are modest at
best, and with a greater downside than any other
cancer we screen for.
 —OTIS BRAWLEY, MD, PROFESSOR OF
 HEMATOLOGY, ONCOLOGY, AND MEDICINE AT
 THE EMORY UNIVERSITY SCHOOL OF MEDICINE
 AND PROFESSOR OF EPIDEMIOLOGY AT EMORY
 UNIVERSITY ROLLINS SCHOOL OF PUBLIC
 HEALTH

Larry King: Are we telling every man over 40 to have
a PSA test?

John McEnroe [whose father survived prostate
cancer]: I think that's what we are telling them.

Larry King: Take the PSA test. Men over 40, it's a
simple little blood test.
 —*LARRY KING LIVE,* AUGUST 23, 2009

Screening for a disease means checking apparently healthy
people for early signs of that disease. The aim is to treat
before the disease progresses to a point where it poses a serious
health threat. Screening tests for many illnesses, including tuber-
culosis, depression, cervical cancer, breast cancer, colon cancer,
skin cancer, and prostate cancer, are commonplace in most mod-
ernized countries. We also screen for risk factors for heart disease,

including high cholesterol, high blood pressure, and high triglyc-erides, and for imbalances in blood sugar that seem set to launch into type 2 diabetes.

In the best case, screening saves lives and prevents suffering. But screening tests for some diseases fail to have a substantial effect on survival. And they may cause more harm than good because they can lead to aggressive treatment of diseases that might not otherwise cause any harm. Allopathic treatments applied to cure early-stage disease may cause side effects that are worse than the disease itself. As you can see from the bat-tling expert opinions headlining this chapter (plus the not-so-expert opinions of a talk show host and a retired tennis player), some believe that this has been the case with the PSA test for prostate cancer.

You've probably already had the PSA, maybe many times. You may be grateful for its role in diagnosing you at an early stage, where you are more or less sure of survival. Or you may be post-treatment, having your PSA monitored with a highly sensi-tive form of this test to look out for recurrence. If you fall into the latter category, you should know that the benefit of PSA testing in those circumstances is not being questioned. It is a very good way to keep an eye out for a recurrence and to con-sider treatment of spreading cancer cells before they manifest into a clinical metastasis.

The issues with the PSA have to do with the initial detection of cancers that are small, slow-growing, and unlikely to ever pose a threat to a man's health. If you are making initial treatment deci-sions about a cancer that may not ever pose a risk to your health, you need to know the PSA story. And even if you aren't, the PSA story is a good illustration of the ways in which modern medicine errs—and a testament to the need for patients to be educated and actively involved in their own treatment.

In modern medicine, we can't grasp whether a screening method is clearly worth the risk until it has been in use for a number of years. We can guess that early detection is better because men who are diagnosed with cancer are more likely to have treatable, curable cancers, and we can decide that large-scale screening is a good idea based on this supposition.

That's what we did with PSA screening once we realized, back in the early 1990s, that about one in four men with a PSA above 4 nanograms per milliliter (ng/ml) turned out to have prostate cancer. Once we spent several years testing and treating millions of people and collecting data, we had enough information to crunch the numbers regarding overall effects on the risk of dying from the disease we're screening for versus threats to quality of life from potentially unnecessary treatments. And we found that for PSA screening, the risk versus benefit equation isn't as straightforward as we'd initially hoped it would be.

Battle of the PSA Recommendations

While one wouldn't necessarily take medical advice from Larry King and John McEnroe, their recommendation to every man over 40 to have the PSA test is based on the guidelines of the American Urological Association. But the AUA's guidelines differ from those created by the American Cancer Society (ACS), which say that men over 50 *might* benefit from the PSA test but that the evidence in its favor is much too weak to merit across-the-board recommendations.

The ACS's 2010 guidelines state that men 50 and up with average risk (no immediate family members with prostate cancer; not African American) should "receive information that allows them to make an informed decision in collaboration with their health care providers" about whether or not to have a PSA test. Men who are not expected to live more than 10 years (owing to advanced age or poor health) do not need to have the test. Men in higher-risk categories are advised to start testing earlier—at 40 or 45 years of age.

PSA Basics

The key concept to keep in mind is that the PSA is *not* a cancer test, it is a prostate test. When PSA shows up beyond a certain level in the bloodstream, the cause *may* be cancer . . . but *it may not be.* An elevated PSA could also indicate several other conditions in the prostate: prostatitis (inflammation of the prostate), benign prostate enlargement, or possibly some kind of trauma to the gland.

Usually, a high PSA is first found by an internist who's doing a general physical on a man. Most internists also use the digital rectal exam (DRE) to try to find any lumps, uneven areas, or hardnesses in the prostate, which can be felt through the wall of the rectum with a gloved, lubricated finger. Traditionally, a PSA above 4 ng/ml and/or a suspicious DRE leads to a referral to a urologist for a prostate biopsy.

Since PSA testing has been clinically available, most physicians have taken on the practice of recommending yearly PSA screening tests to middle-aged men. There is no doubt in my mind that the widespread use of this screening test for prostate cancer has dramatically changed the way this disease is detected, treated, and monitored. There has been a corresponding explosion in the number of cancers detected, and the PSA has definitely helped to diagnose and treat men at far earlier stages of the disease. In fact, for the majority of men diagnosed in 2011, bone or lymph node metastases will be extremely rare, and a CT scan or bone scan will rarely be needed.

Before the prostate-specific antigen test came into widespread use in the 1990s, men were rarely diagnosed with prostate cancer before it had spread. Only 4 percent of men diagnosed with this cancer could be cured. As of the second decade of the second millennium, 5-year survival from prostate cancer is nearly 100 percent.

The flip side of this success story is that this same widespread screening and diagnosis has resulted in a leap in diagnoses of prostate cancer amounting to 30 percent. The greatest increase in diagnoses since 1986, when the PSA test was introduced, occurred in men under 50. *More than seven times* as many men in this age group got the "you have prostate cancer" talk from a physician in the late 2000s than in the mid-1980s—and many have gotten treatments they didn't need and that might have caused permanent, life-changing harm to their reproductive or urinary tract health.

Not all prostate cancers that are diagnosed require medical treatment. Many grow so slowly that they will never reach the point of causing significant illness or death. After years of aggressively treating even the smallest prostate cancers, we now realize that many men who would not have died or even become ill from slow-growing prostate cancers ended up having aggressive treatments that detracted significantly from their quality of life. Someone once said, quite accurately, that "more men die *with* prostate cancer than *from* prostate cancer."

Although prostate surgeries and other treatments have come a long way, about a third of men who undergo treatment for prostate cancer end up impotent or incontinent. One large-scale study published in 2010 found that for every life saved through early detection by PSA screening, four men became impotent and fewer than one man became incontinent. (This figure might seem confusing—how can you have fewer than one man?—but it's sort of like those statistics that talk about families having an average of 2.3 children. It's a figure boiled down from larger numbers.)

In 2009 and 2010, initial results from four very large studies—three American and one European—revealed some troubling information about the value of the PSA as a screening test:

- Two of these studies found that men who had PSA screening actually had increased mortality compared with men who don't. In other words, they were more likely to die during follow-up.

- Another study found no significant difference in longevity between men who were screened and men who were not screened.

- The fourth study (the European one) found that screening substantially improved survival.

One study, which was published in the *Journal of the National Cancer Institute* in 2009, tracked men who had PSA screening between the years of 1986 and 2005. These researchers found that

1,305,600 additional cases of prostate cancer were diagnosed in those years. Of those cases, 1,004,800 received definitive treatment. And the study concluded that those 1.3 million additional diagnoses averted only 56,000 deaths from prostate cancer. That may sound like a worthwhile number of deaths to avert—but consider this conclusion made by the study's authors:

> Using the most optimistic assumption about the benefit of screening—that the entire decline in prostate cancer mortality observed during this period is attributable to these additional diagnoses—for each man who experienced the presumed benefit, more than 20 had to be diagnosed with prostate cancer. . . . The vast majority of those treated did not benefit from early detection.

The European study found that giving PSA tests every 4 years *did* lower the death rate of men from this disease by about 20 percent. The way this pans out: For approximately every 1,000 men screened, 1 man's death from prostate cancer was prevented.

It may be that men who have aggressive cancers that are found with PSA screening are not likely to benefit from early detection, while men with less aggressive cancers found with the PSA ended up having treatments they didn't really need for cancers that almost certainly would not have killed them.

Some other complicating factors: The PSA doesn't always reveal prostate cancer. Men can have a normal PSA and still have the disease—even advanced disease. When the PSA comes back clean despite the existence of prostate cancer, we call this a *false negative*. Obesity, which is a risk factor for aggressive prostate cancer, can mask high PSA because of a higher dilution of the protein in the blood. And even a sky-high PSA doesn't always mean cancer.

As much as the average man would like to believe he's going to live forever, the fact is that life expectancy for an American man is right around 80 years at this writing. If a man is older than 75, and he gets a PSA, and the PSA finds something, the likelihood that any subsequent treatment will prolong his life—or even be worth the side effects—is minuscule. This is why many guidelines now suggest that a man with a life expectancy less than 10 years probably won't benefit from PSA screening. On the other hand, a man 75 or up who has already gone ahead with screening can probably dramatically improve his overall health and quality of life with the holistic chemoprevention program described in Part III of this book. That program carries no risk and promotes health throughout the body, not just urologically.

If men 75 and older have had serial PSAs in the past and there has been no significant rise, it's still unlikely that he'll develop an aggressive form of the disease and die of it. Guidelines still vary pretty dramatically from organization to organization. This is a choice men need to make on their own (hopefully with physician support), taking into account their general state of health and family history.

Putting Personal Testimonies into Perspective

Every time cancer screening guidelines change, lots of people come forward to talk about how they would not have found their cancers in time to undergo successful treatment if they had not had this screening test.

It's hard to watch this kind of personal testimony without feeling affected. It's easier to identify with a human being who has a compelling story to tell than with a bunch of numbers that have undergone rigorous statistical analysis. It's easy to forget that each of those hundreds of thousands of numbers involves the life, health, and longevity of an individual human being and that they matter just as much as that person solicited to go on camera and tell his or her story of catching cancer early. The ones who don't have their lives saved by the screening test just aren't as newsworthy.

As someone who sits and talks with people who have prostate cancer every day I go to work, I know how compelling these stories can be. Every day, patients tell me, "Thank God I had the PSA test, Dr. Katz," or, "Thank God I had that biopsy." They feel that if they had not had these tests and found out that they had prostate cancer, it might have killed them. They've heard stories or know of people who got diagnosed too late or died from prostate cancer.

It's these human stories, these individual anecdotes, that are not discussed in the medical studies. The brilliant statisticians who sit at their desks with complex charts and numbers and graphs don't deal with the emotional aspects of the disease and screening. They can crunch the numbers on millions of men, but what about the man sitting across from me who is anxious because his best friend died of prostate cancer last year and wants to do *everything possible* to avoid going through what his friend did? Maybe he's 70 and has no family history and no urinary symptoms, but he's coming to me because he wants the test. He doesn't care about the statistics; he just needs to know his PSA.

I know how scary this disease is when it progresses to a point where it has to be treated aggressively in order to save a life. But this doesn't change the fact that a test that finds cancer very early may not prevent people from dying from that cancer. And sometimes it creates a tidal wave of overtreatment that does so much harm, the lives saved don't end up meriting that much collateral damage.

The Costs of Overdiagnosis

PSA screening drastically increases the number of men treated for cancers that would never pose any real threat to their health. For every man saved from death by prostate cancer, over 1,000 have to be diagnosed and treated for the disease. While this is great for that one man—and to be honest, that man might be *you*—what about all the other men who dutifully get their screenings and submit to expensive treatments . . . without any benefit to their life span or their overall health and with all the risks such treatments entail?

Although you might be the fellow saved by early detection, you might also be the fellow who comes to me after having unnecessary radiation treatments with a urethra that has become so scarred, it has closed up. You might be the man who ends up impotent from prostate cancer treatments when he didn't really require treatment at all.

The answer here: personalized, individualized treatment and detailed patient education. Medicine has become so complex that doctors have to be willing to personalize therapy. We need to tailor treatments to individual patients. I'll tell you more about how I do that in my own practice in Chapters 6 and 7, and you'll learn in this book how to be an informed patient who can participate in this process with your medical team.

Every day, I see patients in my practice who have been diagnosed with prostate cancer by a urologist and have been given the laundry list of standard options from which they are expected to choose. "Here are your options," the man hears. "Surgery, radiation, cryosurgery, hormones, or do nothing. Call me in a week and let me know."

Of course, most men would rather have the physician's opinion on the best course. "Doctor, what would you suggest I do?" they ask, innocently expecting the doctor to give an unbiased opinion. Most often, these men are told to have either surgery or radiation, depending on the level of expertise of that particular doctor. And if the doctor owns part of the radiation center to which the patient will end up being referred, guess what is almost always recommended? That's right—radiation. This form of medical evaluation is what I consider the "best of the 1990s." The tools we have now to refine diagnosis and treatment plans go way beyond this kind of standard advice.

We need to tailor treatments to individual patients. This requires in-depth discussion with the patient. It's best to include a close family member (spouse, partner, or blood relative) who understands the man's background, lifestyle, any underlying medical illnesses, and sex life.

We all know that unnecessary treatments can be hazardous to a man's health and to the quality of his life, but there is also a substantial economic cost for these treatments. Reducing unneeded biopsies and far more costly allopathic treatments could have a big impact on health care costs. A more conservative, integrative approach to treatment could make a substantial dent in the cost of treating prostate cancer, which at this writing averages more than $42,500 per patient.

What I Recommend

The recommendations I give for PSA screening are to have the test each year after age 50, unless a man has a family history of the disease. If there is a family history, I suggest starting to test at age 40. I do rely on age-specific ranges for the PSA. Those ranges vary slightly depending on the source. However, the patient's physician will have a set range he uses to evaluate his own patients.

The key here is not whether or not to have the PSA. It's the way in which the results of the test are interpreted and acted upon. A single, isolated elevated PSA does not have to mean an immediate biopsy any more than a small cancer has to mean immediate radiation treatment or surgery.

Watchful waiting and chemoprevention aren't the only strategies we have at our disposal here. We don't yet have great medical tools for distinguishing between a slow-growing, relatively unthreatening prostate cancer and one that is likely to be deadly. That's what we most need to develop to make the PSA a more effective screening tool and to avoid overtreatment. For now, here are a few of the principles I use in my practice to try to spare men from having a prostate biopsy unless it's absolutely necessary. If a man comes to me with a high PSA reading, I might:

Repeat the PSA and measure free versus total PSA as well. The PSA protein can exist in several forms in the bloodstream. It can float freely or be bound up to another protein. The ratio of free to bound form can be helpful here when determining the next diagnostic step. Just as there are two forms of cholesterol that impact heart disease risk differently, these two forms of PSA have a different predictive value for prostate cancer. This PSA derivative can be helpful in those patients who have a borderline PSA level for their age.

If free PSA is low, the man is more likely to have prostate cancer.

This helps us decide whether a biopsy is needed. There is some debate over the cutoff point where biopsy is recommended, but generally, if free PSA is below 20 percent, there's a much higher chance of cancer than if free PSA is above 25 percent.

Give a transrectal ultrasound to visualize the prostate gland. Transrectal ultrasound (also known as a sonogram) enables the physician to see the size of a man's prostate. Knowing this information enables me to determine the man's PSA density (PSAD)—the PSA divided by the size of the prostate in grams.

If two men the same age both have a PSA of 8, their likelihood of prostate cancer can be further determined by measuring the size of the gland. Let's say a transrectal sonogram shows me that one man has a 100-gram gland (that's very large!) and the other has a normal gland size of 20 grams. The man with the 20-gram gland is *much* more likely to have prostate cancer, whereas the PSA of the man with the 100-gram gland is more likely to be due to an overabundance of benign tissue.

The lower the PSAD, the lower the chances that prostate cancer is present. A gland with a density greater than 0.15 should be biopsied.

Perform a genetic test designed to identify cancer cells in the prostate. The PCA-3 gene test is relatively new as of this writing. It looks at a specific gene that has been linked to prostate cancer. If the test shows that this gene is "turned on"—what molecular biologists refer to as "overexpressed"—there is a high likelihood of prostate cancer being present in the gland.

To give the PCA-3 test, the urologist first massages the prostate so that some prostate cells are shed into the urine. Then the man gives a urine sample, which is sent to a lab to be tested. A score above 35 on that test strongly suggests that cancer is present and gives me the green light to do a biopsy. In some studies, PCA-3 has

been shown to be better than PSA in predicting the presence of prostate cancer.

Digital Rectal Exam: Also of Questionable Value?

Some evidence suggests that even the digital rectal exam may not be lifesaving. The American Cancer Society's guidelines, as well as those from the American College of Preventive Medicine, don't push the DRE as an important screening tool. But with the DRE, as with the PSA, we can use results not as singular decision-making tools, but as part of a comprehensive diagnostic picture that enables doctor and patient to work together to make reasoned treatment choices—or the choice to delay treatment.

During the DRE, the physician feels the prostate with a gloved, lubricated finger. The patient's job here is to relax as much as possible. Tensing up can make the exam painful. The physician's job is to find any nodules and check for hardness or asymmetry. It is my practice to do a DRE on all patients that are undergoing an evaluation for prostate cancer, or even in those men already treated.

Prostate Biopsy: Everything You Need to Know

If there is a persistently high PSA, or a definite nodule on the rectal exam, the usual next step is to undergo a prostate biopsy under transrectal ultrasound.

Biopsy has changed a good deal since my early years as a urologist. Whereas early biopsies didn't reliably take samples throughout the gland—meaning there was a good chance the biopsy could miss areas that were cancerous—we now use a method that takes numerous samples from throughout the prostate. This increases our chances of visualizing the tissues thoroughly, catching any and all areas of dysplasia or cancer. We can then use those samples to figure out how advanced and how aggressive the cancer cells are.

I'll usually elect to perform a biopsy when a man has:

- frank abnormalities found during the DRE

- a PSA above 2.5, without any explanation for it being elevated (e.g., prostate inflammation or enlargement, or sexual activity or trauma within 24 hours of PSA testing)

- a trend of rising PSA over a period of time (e.g., if three PSA tests done over a year and a half show a rise of at least 0.75 ng/ml per year)

- a doubling of PSA over a period up to 3 years (PSA doubling time less than 3 years)

Both of the latter indicators describe *PSA velocity*—the speed of change in PSA over time. At this writing, however, Memorial Sloan-Kettering Cancer Center has conducted a large research study (involving 5,519 men) that brought the use of PSA velocity into question as a diagnostic tool. Researchers found that men who were given PSA velocity tests to see whether they needed biopsy had a one-in-seven chance of receiving a biopsy, while only 1 in 20 men judged on PSA alone ended up having this procedure. This suggests that using PSA velocity to decide whether a man needs a biopsy may contribute to overdiagnosis and overtreatment.

For the privilege of having numerous holes poked in his prostate gland, followed by a highly anxious period spent waiting for results, a man (or his insurer) can expect to fork over about $1,200.

Unfortunately, there is a profit motive in this for some physicians. Biopsies represent a significant revenue stream for urologists. They aren't generally considered to be harmful—they can certainly be justified under the "better safe than sorry" directive—but they can and do lead to overtreatment and unnecessary expense. There's just no way around this fact. Cancer is big business. This is a good thing to keep in mind as you consider whether a biopsy is right for you. Have a repeat PSA first, as well as a urine test to make sure there is no infection present.

If you do end up having a biopsy, your urologist will probably have you clean out your bowels with an enema either at home or in the office beforehand. This will make testing easier for the physician and will reduce your chances of infection following the procedure.

You will also likely be advised to take a week off of any medications that thin the blood (NSAIDs like aspirin, ibuprofen, or naproxen; Coumadin, Plavix, or other blood thinners) and blood-thinning supplements like vitamin E and fish oil. The risk of excess bleeding following a biopsy is low, but it's best to give the body its full clotting power just in case.

For 1 day before the procedure and 3 days following, I usually have patients take a quinolone antibiotic (Levaquin) to further avoid the possibility of infection at the biopsy site. With a pre-biopsy enema and antibiotic therapy, the likelihood of developing infection is less than 2 percent. I also make sure there is no urinary tract infection before the procedure. Most urologists will also give an antibiotic by injection just before performing the biopsy.

To relieve any pain associated with biopsy, doctors administer a pain-relieving nerve block, using an ultrasound probe to guide a small needle that injects numbing medication into the wall of the rectum where samples will be taken. Modern ultrasound probes are very narrow and don't usually cause discomfort.

Once the numbing medication kicks in, the biopsy can begin. Samples are generally taken transrectally, through the wall of the rectum, using the ultrasound probe to visualize the gland. Most urologists use a biopsy tool that has (unfortunately) come to be called a biopsy gun—it is loaded with a small, very fine needle, which is "shot"into the prostate about 2 inches. It then pops right back out into the tool, and the tissue in the needle's hollow core is placed into a specimen container. This process is repeated up to 12 times.

Some doctors will take fewer than 12 cores, but the biopsy will be more accurate if more cores are extracted. Before you lie down on the table, ask your urologist how many cores he plans to take. If he intends to take fewer than 12, ask why and let him know you know that more cores means a more accurate diagnosis. Following a biopsy, traces of blood may show up in the urine for a few days and in semen for several weeks.

With information from a biopsy—or from the PSA and other tests that suggest prostate disease but may not indicate that biopsy is necessary—you're ready to move into the next phase. In rare cases, a biopsy will miss cancer that actually does exist in the prostate gland. If a man has a negative biopsy but his PSA continues to rise, a repeat biopsy may be called for. For some men who are found to have cancer, this might mean surgery, radiation, or hormone therapy. For others, active holistic surveillance may be all that's needed. The decision to do one or the other is an intensely personal one that ultimately needs to be made between the medical team, patient, and patient's loved ones.

In chapters to come, you'll learn in depth about the risks, benefits, and indications for treatments and surveillance. Keep in mind that the holistic steps recommended in Chapters 8 to 10 will benefit every man—from the man who needs no treatment to the man who decides that surgery to remove the prostate gland is his best course of action.

CHAPTER 5

STAGING TESTS FOR PROSTATE CANCER

Biopsy results will come back within about 5 business days, possibly sooner. The typical biopsy report includes a variety of information that in combination enables your medical team to either rule out cancer or *stage* your cancer. Staging is the process of determining how advanced, aggressive, and risky the cancer is. We use this information to determine the course of treatment.

Here's what you'll find in the results of your biopsy:

- Information about the number of samples and appearance of the tissue, also known as a gross description. This may include description of the color and consistency of the samples.

- A description of the cells in the samples as perceived by the pathologist. Cancerous cells may be described as adenocarcinoma. Cells that are abnormal but not cancerous are described as prostatic intraepithelial neoplasia or atypical small acinar proliferation.

- Gleason grading of the cancerous cells. This is a score given to rate how different cancerous cells are from surrounding tissue, which tells us how aggressive the cancer is likely to be. The lowest grade is a 2 and the highest is a 10. The higher the Gleason score, the more important it is to treat the cancer promptly. Once your biopsy has discovered cancer, more testing options may follow. These tests are designed to give your urological team as solid an idea as possible of the location and extent of what we're dealing with. When added to what's learned from biopsy—which is conveyed in the form of a Gleason score—this information helps us to make the most precise treatment choices for each patient. It offers us the best chances for avoiding overtreatment while giving the most effective treatment possible to each individual patient. In this chapter, you'll learn which tests are most helpful and what kind of information they're likely to yield.

Clinical Tumor Staging

In this part of the process, your medical team will use various tests to figure out where cancer is located in your body. The most important question to answer is whether the cancer is isolated to the prostate gland, within the tough capsule that surrounds the gland. If it has spread outside the gland, surgical interventions are unlikely to be an option.

All of these tests—the biopsy, the PSA, and the other tests described in the preceding chapter—can yield worthwhile information, or they can yield *false positives* or *false negatives*. A false positive is a test result that seems to reveal disease or more advanced disease when none is present. A false negative is a test result that fails to reveal disease where it *does* exist. No test is infallible, but the tools we have for staging today are as good as they've ever been.

Bone Scan Testing

To determine whether prostate cancer has spread to the bone—usually its first destination if it does spread—we perform a radionuclide bone scan. You'll go to a hospital or testing center to have this scan. A special material with low-level radioactivity is infused into your body through an intravenous (IV) line; this substance is attracted to areas where bone tissue is damaged. Once the radioactive agent has settled—this takes a couple of hours—the next step is to have the actual scan, where you lie on a table while a camera puts together a picture of your whole skeleton. Areas where bone is damaged show up as "hot spots" on the final scan. Since damage can be caused by cancer, arthritis, or other bone diseases, these hot spots aren't conclusive evidence of cancer having spread to the bone. Other tests, like bone biopsies, CT scans, or MRI scans, help determine whether these areas of bone are affected by cancer or by something else.

Over the course of a few days after this test, the radioactive material exits the body through urine. Ask your doctor whether any precautions need to be taken to prevent exposure of loved ones to this material.

CT (Computerized Tomography) Scan

This special X-ray makes a detailed cross-sectional image of whatever part of the body we're interested in examining. It rotates around the body, creating image "slices" that are then compiled by a computer program into a cross section of the body part in question. The CT scan is most commonly prescribed when it appears that cancer is likely to have spread outside the prostate. It allows your medical team to see which organs and/or lymph nodes may be affected. A CT scan isn't helpful for evaluating early-stage prostate cancer that is unlikely to have spread.

You'll be asked to drink enough liquid to fill your bladder before the test. A full bladder helps push the large intestine away from the prostate, which helps with better visibility for the scan. Before the test, you may also be given an IV containing contrast solution, which helps make a clearer CT image. Some people feel flushed or have allergic reactions in response to the contrast solution. If you have had allergic reactions during medical tests before, or if you have significant allergies in general, let your doctor know before you get the contrast solution.

The CT scan itself takes only a few minutes. Results can be read immediately; ask your doctor how long you can expect to wait to get your results.

MRI (Magnetic Resonance Imaging) Scan

MRI is another option used to look at cancer that is likely to have spread outside of the prostate gland. Instead of using X-rays to see into the body, the MRI scan uses strong magnets and radio waves, which enter the body and emerge again in a pattern that can be "read" by your medical team. Magnets can disrupt the function of pacemakers or other medical implants; people who rely upon these kinds of devices may not be able to have MRI testing. An MRI scan can paint a crystal-clear picture of the prostate and surrounding tissues and organs (the seminal vesicles, the bladder). When the MRI is being done to evaluate prostate cancer, an endorectal coil (a special probe) may be inserted into the patient's rectum to improve the accuracy of the scan.

When having an MRI, you will be expected to lie down inside a narrow tube and stay still for up to an hour while the machine clicks, buzzes, and whirrs. Headphones with music may be provided for those who don't like enclosed spaces.

Results of an MRI can take anywhere from 3 days to 2 weeks to come back.

ProstaScint Scan

The ProstaScint is another way of scanning the body to check for any spread of prostate cancer. It's not a very accurate test, and most urologists use it rarely, if at all. I generally order this test only for men who have already undergone treatment for prostate cancer, in order to zero in on the site of potential recurrences when the PSA starts to rise. The ProstaScint uses mildly radioactive material that is attracted specifically to both cancerous and non-cancerous prostate cells—not just in bones, but anywhere in the body, including organs and lymph nodes.

If you have this test, you'll receive an injection of the ProstaScint agent. About a half hour later, you'll lie down while a specialized camera creates an image of your body. The scan is usually repeated 3 to 5 days later, and results will be available within a few days after the second scan.

Lymph Node Biopsy

If your medical team has good reason to believe your cancer has spread beyond the prostate to surrounding lymph nodes, a biopsy of those nodes might be deemed necessary. These procedures (also known as lymph node dissection, lymphadenectomy, or lymph node biopsy) may be done in a few different ways:

- Surgically: Lymph nodes may be removed for biopsy through an incision in the lower abdomen. This may be done during open prostatectomy (surgery where the prostate is removed through an incision). When lymph nodes are removed during prostatectomy, they are sent with the gland to be examined by a pathologist to help dictate the next stages of treatment. When the PSA is above 20 ng/ml and the Gleason score from the biopsy is over 7, the surgeon may have a pathologist look at the lymph nodes surrounding the prostate during surgery before deciding whether to remove the gland. It may not be worth the risk to remove the prostate if the cancer has already spread to the lymph nodes.

- Laparoscopically: A laparoscope is a slender tube with a very small video camera on the end. It can be inserted through an incision as narrow as the width of a single finger. Along with surgical instruments inserted through other small incisions, it enables the surgeon to remove lymph nodes around the prostate with a procedure that may require only 1 to 2 days' healing time. Any scars left by laparoscopic procedures are very small. This isn't a common route with prostate cancer, but it may be done in patients who are not opting for surgery and are instead considering radiation.

- With fine needle aspiration: Some radiologists are trained to perform this procedure on patients whose lymph nodes look enlarged on a CT or MRI scan. The scan image helps the radiologist guide a very thin needle through the lower abdomen and into the affected node to take a sample of tissue. A local anesthesia is used to make this procedure painless.

Prostate Cancer Staging

Once your medical team has performed all the needed tests, a complete picture of the prostate cancer's stage can be drawn for the purpose of determining a prognosis (how the disease is expected to progress) and a treatment plan.

Prognostic classification is most often done through a categorization known as TNM. T (tumor) is an evaluation of the size of the primary tumor. N (node) describes how much regional lymph node involvement has been detected. M (metastasis) is an evaluation of distant metastasis—whether the cancer has spread to other parts of the body. The Gleason grade, which describes the actual appearance of the cells and their potential to do damage in the body, is also used to create this complete picture.

T Categories: Tumor Growth

The T categories are classified as follows: T1, which breaks down into subcategories of T1a, T1b, and T1c; T2, which breaks down into T2a, T2b, and T2c; T3, which breaks down into T3a and T3b; and T4.

Stage T1: The cancer cells found do not differ much from normal prostate cells. No tumor can be found with transrectal ultrasound. Nothing is felt at all on the DRE.

T1a: Prostate cancer cells are found in tissue removed for other reasons, such as BPH. Cancer is found in less than 5 percent of the tissue that was removed.

T1b: Same as T1a, except that cancer is found in more than 5 percent of removed tissue.

T1c: Cancer is found by needle biopsy that was performed because of a rising PSA.

Stage T2: More of the gland is involved, and the DRE reveals a lump, hardness, or other suggestion of cancer. The cancer appears confined to the prostate.

T2a: Cancer is found in only one-half or less of only one side of the prostate.

T2b: Cancer is found in more than one-half of only one side of the prostate.

T2c: Cancer is found in both halves of the prostate.

Stage T3: Cancer has spread outside of the prostate and may involve the seminal vesicles.

T3a: Cancer has spread beyond the prostate, but not into the seminal vesicles.

T3b: Cancer has spread to the seminal vesicles.

Stage T4: Cancer has spread to invade nearby organs or lymph nodes, possibly including the urethral sphincter (the muscle that helps control the flow of urine), rectum, or pelvic wall.

N Categories: Regional Lymph Node Involvement

This is a simple categorization: Has cancer spread to the lymph nodes in the pelvis or not? If the score is N0, the answer is no—the cancer has not affected pelvic lymph nodes. If it's N1, these nodes are affected.

M Categories: Metastasis

Categories M0, M1, and M1a to M1c describe how far—if at all—the cancer has spread beyond regional lymph nodes.

Stage M0: Cancer has not spread beyond regional lymph nodes.

Stage M1: Cancer has spread beyond regional nodes.

M1a: Cancer has spread to lymph nodes outside the pelvis—also known as distant lymph nodes.

M1b: Cancer has spread to the bones.

M1c: Cancer has spread to other organs, such as brain, lungs, or liver; may or may not have spread to the bones.

Stage Groupings

Once T, N, and M categories are determined, we combine this information with what's known from the Gleason score and the PSA to arrive at something called a stage grouping. A stage grouping is expressed as a Roman numeral. Stage I is least advanced and IV is most advanced.

Now What?

If you have been diagnosed with prostate cancer and undergone staging tests, understanding the results is just the beginning. Each stage has its own prognosis and treatment options, which will be addressed in detail in coming chapters. Take a deep breath and know that you've got a very good chance of getting through this.

Now, let's turn to treatment options.

STAGE I	STAGE IIA	STAGE IIB	STAGE III
One of the following applies:	One of the following applies:	One of the following applies:	T3, N0, M0, any Gleason score, any PSA
T1, N0, M0, Gleason score 6 or less, PSA <10	T1, N0, M0, Gleason score of 7, PSA <20	T2c, N0, M0, any Gleason score, any PSA	**STAGE IV**
OR:	OR:	OR:	One of the following applies:
T2a, N0, M0, Gleason score 6 or less, PSA <10	T1, N0, M0, Gleason score of 6 or less, PSA at least 10 but <20	T1 or T2, N0, M0, any Gleason score, PSA of 20 or more	T4, N0, M0, any Gleason score, any PSA
	OR:	OR:	OR:
	T2a or T2b, N0, M0, Gleason score of 7 or less, PSA <20	T1 or T2, N0, M0, Gleason score of 8 or higher, any PSA	Any T, N1, M0, any Gleason score, any PSA
			OR:
			Any T, any N, M1, any Gleason score, any PSA

CHAPTER 6

NOT YOUR FATHER'S PROSTATE CANCER TREATMENTS: THE TRUTH ABOUT MAINSTREAM MEDICAL THERAPY FOR PROSTATE CANCER

Informed by the results of diagnostic and staging tests, your urological team now has all the information needed to figure out a treatment plan and offer you several options.

In this chapter, I'll tell you what you need to know about these options before making decisions with your medical team. Before you begin this journey, remember that there are always multiple options when it comes to prostate cancer treatment and that you should never feel you have to act right away. And for most men there's no such thing as only one "right" option. Watchful waiting, radical surgery, hormone ablation therapy, radiation, cryosurgery, HIFU, and robotic surgery are all options for early-stage, localized disease.

When cancer is detected at an early stage, it is usually small and slow-growing. I believe that watchful waiting (also known as active surveillance) may be your best option under these circumstances. I exhort all readers who are considering this approach to employ the holistic and chemopreventive strategies described in Chapters 8 through 10. I'll explain in those chapters how these strategies can be used to delay cancer's growth. Their effect may be powerful enough to make surgery, radiation, or hormone drugs unnecessary at any point for readers with these slow-growing types of cancer.

Even if more aggressive treatment seems called for, the chances men have of going through these treatments without becoming impotent or incontinent are much better than they once were. Exciting progress has been made in the area of minimally invasive prostate surgeries—in particular, laparoscopic surgeries performed through tiny incisions. Robots, lasers, and other advanced technologies used in these procedures help patients avoid side effects and maintain an excellent quality of life.

This chapter covers, in detail (and in plain English), the potential benefits and hazards of each mainstream treatment. Which treatment is right for you? Together with your medical team, you'll consider the grade and stage of your disease, your age and general state of health, and the likelihood of side effects. You'll be asked to carefully consider your willingness to risk the side effects in question. And you'll learn what to expect before, during, and after each type of therapy, including the chances (according to the research) that you'll experience a recurrence.

If you go into a physician's office without the information in this chapter, you stand a good chance of being rushed into choosing to treat with either surgery or radiation. Armed with the knowledge in this chapter, you'll be far less befuddled when you enter this difficult conversation with your doctors.

Active Holistic Surveillance

According to urology researcher Laurence Klotz, early-stage prostate cancer is not even exactly cancer as it is generally defined. In an article published on the Web site of the Prostate Cancer Canada Network, he writes: "Part of the problem is that, for some men who are detected at an early stage, the word cancer is almost a misnomer. . . . Cancer implies rampaging disease, but in most cases of early stage prostate cancer, that's not the case."

The word *cancer* has frightening implications, and those implications lead many patients to a seek-and-destroy mind-set. Physicians may also hold this mind-set, along with a notion that it's better to overtreat than take a chance of undertreating. With some cancers this attitude makes sense, but with a generally slow-growing form of the disease like prostate cancer, it's safe in many cases to choose not to go after the cancer aggressively. In certain cases of these early-stage, low-risk cancers, what I usually recommend is active *holistic* surveillance, which incorporates the nutritional and lifestyle changes described in later chapters.

From here on, if you read the words *active surveillance* in this book, know that I'm referring to the holistic version. I won't use the term *watchful waiting* from this point forward, because it generally indicates a more passive approach than active surveillance. Peter Carroll, a urologist and researcher at the University of California at San Francisco, put it this way in an interview with journalist Andrew Schorr: "I always say watchful waiting was not enough watching and too much waiting . . . there was a time when some men were not treated and followed not very carefully and only treated when they developed metastatic disease, disease in the bone usually, and then they were treated with hormonal therapy."

Are you a candidate for active surveillance? I believe the answer is "yes" if:

- You have a PSA below 10 and a Gleason score under 7; and

- Disease is staged at T1 or T2; and

- MRI shows no cancer growth outside your prostate gland; and

- Cancer is not palpable in the DRE (or, if it is palpable, it seems confined to the prostate); and

- Biopsy shows fewer than 4 of at least 12 cores to be positive for cancer; and

- Less than half of any core taken is cancerous.

In the past, older and sicker men have been more likely to get a recommendation to watch and wait, because the risks of treatment are unlikely to pan out as benefits for men whose life expectancy is less than 10 years. But with today's more precise tools for staging, younger men may also have a viable option to defer treatment and track the disease. Even if these younger men end up requiring treatment, they may be able to defer it for many years with active holistic surveillance. Recent data show that even waiting to start mainstream treatments for up to 3 years won't lead to any adverse effects in men who are good candidates for active holistic surveillance.

Since 2002, Dr. Klotz has led a group of Canadian researchers in following a cohort of about 300 men who chose to enroll in the START (Surveillance Therapy Against Radical Treatment) study, which compares treatment of early-stage prostate cancer with active surveillance. The plan is to follow each patient for 20 years, but at this writing data are already available, and they look promising. Average PSA doubling time for these men is 7 years; close to half (42 percent) saw their PSAs double only after a full decade following diagnosis. (Recall that PSA doubling rate shows us how fast the cancer may be growing; a doubling within 18 months or less is considered cause for more aggressive treatment.) Only 5 percent turned out to have faster-growing cancers, where PSA doubled in only a year or less. Nine and a half years into the study, 99.5 percent of the men were still alive.

Active holistic surveillance involves:

- Changes in diet, including reduction or elimination of red meat and dairy

- Dietary supplements, including herbal anti-inflammatories, omega-3 fatty acid supplements, and vitamin D

- A reasonable exercise program (aerobic exercise three times a week)

- Some method of stress reduction, such as yoga and/or meditation

- PSA testing every 3 to 4 months and a repeat DRE at least every 6 months

- A repeat biopsy at 12 to 24 months, even in cases where the PSA is stable, to ensure that cancer volume has not increased and that the Gleason score does not need to be upgraded

If active holistic surveillance seems to demonstrate that the cancer isn't growing, or is growing so slowly that it is not likely to ever cause major problems, the intervals between bouts of testing may be lengthened. This is something to be worked out between doctor and patient.

Prostatectomy: An Overview

If cancer is isolated to the prostate gland but appears to be aggressive enough to merit intervention, surgery and radiation are standard options that should be considered. Let's look first at the different surgical methods used for prostatectomy, which involves removal of the entire prostate, parts of the vas deferentia and seminal vesicles, and (usually) several of the lymph nodes surrounding the gland. I'll cover other surgical procedures where cancerous areas of the prostate are targeted without removing the whole gland—including cryosurgery—in the next section.

So far, studies show that no prostate removal surgery is clearly superior in terms of rates of success (eradicating cancer) and long-term survival. Each procedure has its champions who cite studies supporting their perspective on which surgery is the best. Risks of complications and side effects differ among procedures.

The most important predictor of a good outcome isn't which of these surgeries you choose; it's the skill and experience of the surgeon. Research suggests that the surgeon's experience is the most important variable in terms of a good prostatectomy outcome. If you require surgery, do the legwork necessary to find a center highly experienced in performing the procedure you'll be having. The more times the surgeon who operates on you has done the surgery in question, the more likely you are to have a good result.

The really telling thing about a surgeon's skill is the number of procedures he or she has performed successfully. If you're going to allow someone to remove your prostate, it should be someone who has performed that procedure at least 50 times—preferably over 100 times.

Of the four current surgical options for prostatectomy, two are more invasive, which means that they require open incisions, and two are minimally invasive, which means that they are done via laparoscopy, through very small incisions that heal rapidly.

- *Radical retropubic prostatectomy* (RRP): The prostate is removed through an incision in the belly.

- *Radical perineal prostatectomy* (RPP): The incision is made in the perineum (the space between anus and scrotum).

- *Laparoscopic radical prostatectomy* (LRP): The surgeon uses laparoscopic tools.

- *Robot-assisted laparoscopic radical prostatectomy* (RALP): The surgeon performs laparoscopic surgery with the aid of a highly technologically advanced robotic system, the da Vinci Surgical System.

In 2003, only 9.2 percent of prostatectomies were minimally invasive. By 2007, robotic prostatectomy comprised 43.2 percent of prostate removal surgeries. And at the start of 2011, it was estimated that over 75 percent of radical prostatectomies would be performed using the robot over the course of that year. Of course, this brings into question the possibility that the medical community is overusing its high-tech tools at the expense of patients: Do all of these men really need surgery, or might some benefit more from a different intervention?

As perineal prostatectomy is rarely used today—it carries a relatively high risk of impotence compared with other procedures—we won't dedicate further space to it here.

Before any of these surgical procedures, you'll have a battery of blood tests to rule out any conditions that increase your risk of surgical complications. For 7 to 10 days before your operation, you'll be advised to refrain from taking aspirin or NSAIDs, as they can thin the blood and increase the risk of bleeding during surgery. Also, stop taking any nutritional supplements, especially fish oils, about a week before the procedure.

If you are taking any blood-thinning medications (the most commonly used are Coumadin and Plavix), they will also need to be stopped at least a week prior to surgery—and make sure the surgeon knows about your medication history. In the weeks before surgery, some doctors may advise patients to give a few pints of blood that can then be stored in case a transfusion is needed during the operation. This isn't really necessary; blood transfusions from donors to the blood bank are safe. One of the major advantages of the robotic procedure over the open technique is the much lower risk of requiring a transfusion; in fact, some centers report a less than 5 percent likelihood that a transfusion will be needed following robotic surgery.

You may get instructions for cleaning out the bowels in the day or so before surgery, and you'll be told not to eat for at least 12 hours before going into the operating room.

During all three types of radical prostatectomy, *lymph node dissection*—removal of the lymph nodes surrounding the prostate—may be performed. Some surgeons will immediately have these nodes biopsied to check for any spread of the cancer; this is called a frozen section analysis. The frozen section is done primarily for men with high-risk, high-volume disease because it can help confirm removal of the prostate. In some cases, if cancer is found in the lymph nodes, the surgery may not continue. Removal of the prostate gland is unlikely to effect a cure once cancer spreads outside the gland, and the threat of surgical side effects outweighs the benefit of removing the gland once prostate cancer has spread into the nodes. Other surgeons will remove the lymph nodes with the prostate but will not have the nodes biopsied until after the surgery—so the gland will come out regardless of what's found in those nodes afterward. Since most prostate cancers are found so early, metastasis to the lymph nodes is rarely found during prostatectomy, so the way in which your surgeon deals with the nodes probably won't be a concern for you.

In the PSA era, where cancer is detected by a blood test alone and is considered low-risk based on subsequent tests, the likelihood of finding disease in the nodes is less than 1 percent. In recent years, surgeons have begun to default to leaving lymph nodes alone in these patients. It's important to discuss this aspect of surgery with your doctor beforehand so that you know what to expect. Removing lymph nodes usually does not cause harm, but there can be risks like bleeding, infection, or the development of a *lymphocele*, a collection of lymphatic fluid near an area where the nodes were removed. Rarely, these lymphoceles can get infected or cause the legs to swell. They may need to be drained by an interventional radiologist.

In all three surgeries, general anesthesia is recommended. Radical retropubic prostatectomy patients may be offered spinal or epidural anesthesia, which allows them to be awake during the surgery, but this is a rarely used option.

The three prostatectomy methods described in the table on pages 98 to 101 have similar, excellent rates of success in terms of disease-free, progression-free survival. This will vary according to your own case, of course, and ongoing PSA monitoring is important for every man who has a prostatectomy to ensure that any recurrence is caught early.

Impotence following Prostatectomy: A Realistic Perspective

Before we look at surgical options in detail, let's talk a little about one of the most feared surgical side effects: impotence. Most men are strongly invested in choosing the treatment course least likely to cause impotence, but looking at the statistics on different procedures can be less than informative. What's a man to think about a statistic like the one reported by the National Prostate Cancer Institute—that "51 to 96 percent of patients are affected by impotence" following a radical prostatectomy? Somewhere between half of the men and nearly *all* of the men who have this surgery end up impotent? Where do these numbers come from, and how can a man prepare for what might happen to him based on such wildly varying estimates of risk?

In her excellent article on the subject, *New York Times* health columnist Tara Parker-Pope asks how one study can say that 97 percent of men who had their prostates removed surgically remained potent, while another states that only half of the men who've undergone the same procedures feel their sex lives have returned to normal in the year after surgery. Parker-Pope explains:

> Most top surgeons report that an overwhelming majority of their patients can achieve erections "adequate for intercourse" after the operation. (Candidates for surgery often shop on the Internet for the surgeons who post the best scores.) Under that definition, a man who had regular sex after surgery, a man who managed to have sex only once and a man who struggled mightily each time he had sex would all be considered success stories.
>
> "That definition is misleading," said Dr. Jason D. Engel, director of the urologic robotic surgery program at the George Washington University Hospital. "It doesn't mean it was good intercourse, and it doesn't even mean your penis was hard. That man is going to say, 'I'm impotent.' But in the surgeon's eyes, that man had an erection adequate for intercourse."

If erectile nerves do not appear to be affected by cancer, nerve-sparing surgery is possible, which yields better rates of potency and continence as long as a highly experienced surgeon is doing the surgery. Even if only one of the two nerve bundles responsible for erection can be preserved, a good potency outcome is more likely.

Even with nerve-sparing surgeries, prostatectomy carries a real risk of changing a man's sex life for the worse. Men who have better sexual function before surgery and who are younger are likely to have a better outcome in this regard after surgery. There's no doubt that men under 60 years old with excellent sexual function are more likely (but not guaranteed) to have the same erectile function after surgery as they did before surgery, as long as the erectile nerve bundles are spared by the surgeon. A supportive partner helps, too. But no one is immune from this side effect of prostatectomy. Parker-Pope's article quotes Dr. Andrew McCullough, director of the Sexual Health and Male Infertility and Microsurgery Program in the Department of Urology at the NYU Cancer Institute, who states that "less than 5 percent of patients are as good

Comparison of Prostatectomy Methods

	RADICAL RETROPUBIC PROSTATECTOMY (RRP)	
How it's done	Removal of the prostate gland, seminal vesicles, and part of the vas deferentia through 4–6 cm vertical incision between navel and pubic bone. Sometimes called open prostatectomy.	

[potency-wise] as they were before surgery . . . the one thing you're going to be facing, regardless of what people tell you, is erectile dysfunction (ED). But the good news is that it is eminently treatable. If you accept the fact that you're going to have it, and you address it early on, you shouldn't skip a beat."

This is good advice for doctors and patients alike: Be realistic about the likelihood of this side effect, and be prepared to take steps to rehabilitate penile function following surgery. Many urologists recommend regularly taking erectile dysfunction drugs or using vacuum pump or intracavernosal injections (drugs injected through a very fine needle that bring on erection) soon

LAPAROSCOPIC RADICAL PROSTATECTOMY (LRP)	ROBOT-ASSISTED LAPARASCOPIC PROSTATECTOMY (RALP)
Removal of the prostate gland, seminal vesicles, and part of the vas deferentia performed with laparoscopic tools, which are inserted through several 5–10 mm skin openings. A small camera (endoscope) is also inserted through one of these openings. The abdominal wall is inflated slightly with carbon dioxide to make space to do the surgery. A video monitor shows the surgeon the action going on at the surgery site. Once it has been disconnected, the prostate is removed through a small incision made above the pubic bone.	Removal of the prostate gland, seminal vesicles, and part of the vas deferentia performed with laparoscopic tools, which are inserted through several 5–10 mm skin openings. A small camera (endoscope) is also inserted through one of these openings. The abdominal wall is inflated slightly with carbon dioxide to make space to perform the surgery. The surgeon is assisted by a specialized robot, the da Vinci Surgical System (Intuitive Surgical, Inc., Sunnyvale, California); he or she sits at a remote console and looks into goggles that show a 3-D view of the prostate and surrounding structures. Operating from this console, the surgeon is able to replicate movements by using the robotic arms inside the patient's body.

continued

Comparison of Prostatectomy Methods *(cont.)*

	RADICAL RETROPUBIC PROSTATECTOMY (RRP)	
How long it takes	1.5–3 hours	
Advantages, disadvantages, impact on potency and continence	Slightly higher likelihood of complications related to open surgery: infection, embolism (blood clot formation), pneumonia, lymphocele (a pocket of fluid that accumulates after lymph node removal), and anastomotic stricture (where the reattachment of urethra to bladder becomes constricted). High (40 percent or lower) chance of some degree of urinary incontinence; 51–96 percent have some level of impotence. Risk of impotence is greater in men who had poor erectile function before surgery. One study performed in a center that did high volumes of these surgeries found that 86 percent of men were potent 18 months after nerve-sparing RRP surgery; less busy centers had much lower potency rates Continence rates are consistently high in studies of nerve-sparing surgery, ranging from 85 to 100 percent. When RRP is used to treat localized prostate cancer that has not responded to radiation therapy, the likelihood of urinary incontinence is higher.	
Time in hospital	2–3 days	
Time with catheter	7–14 days; a surgical drain may also be needed for several days at the incision site.	
Recovery period	For 6 weeks following surgery, do not resume exercise program or other physical activity, including lifting anything heavier than 10 pounds.	

LAPAROSCOPIC RADICAL PROSTATECTOMY (LRP)	ROBOT-ASSISTED LAPARASCOPIC PROSTATECTOMY (RALP)
3–8 hours (it's a more challenging procedure to perform than open prostatectomy)	2.5–3 hours
Less invasive than RRP; shorter healing time; less risk of bleeding during surgery. Surgery can take a very long time if surgeon is inexperienced (fewer than 50 surgeries using laparoscopic method). Greater risk of injury to the bowel or bladder than in open prostatectomy. In a 2003 study of 300 men, 81 percent of those under 60 who had nerve-sparing LRP maintained their potency. This figure was lower (53 percent) when all ages were incorporated into the analysis. This same study found that nighttime urinary continence returns slightly faster with laparoscopic surgery than with open surgery.	Requires less training for urologists to achieve good results. The da Vinci robot guides the procedure with improved accuracy, and surgeon has better control and visibility compared with older laparoscopic procedure. At this writing, RALP is performed much more often than LRP. Still, experience matters; successful outcomes with good continence and potency results are more likely with surgeons who do a lot of robotic prostatectomies. A study published in 2009 of 1,938 men who had minimally invasive surgery and 6,899 men who had open prostatectomy found that while surgical complications like transfusions were lower with RALP, the chance of genitourinary complications after RALP was roughly twice that of open surgery. Likelihood of urinary incontinence and impotence in men who had RALP was slightly higher than in men who had open surgery.
2 days	1–2 days
7 days	7 days
For 2–4 weeks following surgery, do not resume exercise program or other physical activity, including lifting anything heavier than 10 pounds.	For 2–4 weeks following surgery, do not resume exercise program or other physical activity, including lifting anything heavier than 10 pounds.

after surgery to improve blood flow to the penis, even before sexual activity resumes. I'll give you more information about this later in the chapter, but I do agree that early penile rehabilitation is key for a successful outcome.

Even when erectile function is reduced following surgery, sensation in the penis remains, as does the ability to have an orgasm—although without a prostate gland and seminal vesicles, orgasms will be "dry," with no discharge of semen. And because surgical removal of the prostate removes a section of the urethra, some men experience a slight reduction in penile length following surgery. Both changes may take some getting used to, but they aren't enough to ruin the experience for men who really want to have a satisfying sex life after surgery.

Besides, research shows that improvements in both continence and potency can occur even 2 or more years following surgery. It may be a slow road back for some men, but positive changes can happen even when they don't happen in the first year. Sexual function may continue to improve for up to 4 years after prostate removal surgery.

Once removed, the prostate gland is thoroughly examined by a pathologist. Should the results of that examination reveal new information, you'll discuss that with your medical team and decide whether additional treatments might be called for.

The pathology report is a detailed analysis that describes margin status, final Gleason score, extent of the cancer, and the presence or absence of any disease outside of the prostate capsule. These results are very important and can determine the need for additional therapy (aside from surgery) as well as the likelihood that prostate cancer will not come back. When there is no evidence of any cancer outside of the prostate (so-called organ-confined cancer), the man is said to have a surgical cure. This man has a greater than 90 percent chance of having undetectable PSA at 6 weeks postsurgery and of having that PSA will remain undetectable for 5 years.

Following any prostate removal surgery, you will need to have a urinary catheter for anywhere from 3 days to over a week. All prostatectomies involve cutting the urethra from where it enters the prostate gland and then reattaching it to the bladder. Time is required for this reattachment to heal. A surgical drain is also left in place following all three types of prostate surgery; the drain is stitched in place and can usually be removed the following day if there is no significant drainage in the tubing.

Urinary continence may take some time to return after surgery—1 to 3 months is not abnormal—and nocturnal (nighttime) continence may take longer to return than daytime continence. After catheter removal, retrain the urinary muscles by urinating whenever you feel the urge.

Do Kegel exercises every day: Contract and release the sphincter muscles as though you were going to urinate, then stop the flow of urine. If you can do 300 or so repetitions a day, your continence is likely to return more quickly. I suggest doing Kegels in the weeks before surgery as well.

Penile Rehabilitation following Prostatectomy

Following prostate surgery, I encourage men to take an active role in restoring sexual function. Much of this is about maintaining adequate blood flow and oxygen to the penis with erectile dysfunction medications (Viagra, Levitra, Cialis) or other methods. Some men are not good candidates for oral ED drugs owing to heart problems or the use of certain medications that can create harmful interactions. Other methods like vacuum pumps or intracavernosal injections of a drug called alprostadil are better options for these men. Rather than using ED-reversing methods just for intercourse, men are advised to use them on a regular schedule during the recovery period. This helps keep erectile tissues healthy while nerves that control erection recover from the trauma of prostate removal.

During my residency training, we used to tell patients they'd have to wait a year after prostate surgery for their erections to return to normal. This is no longer the case. Many leading authorities in the field agree that early restoration of blood flow strongly supports long-term satisfaction with erections. The blood that enters the penis is rich in oxygen, which prevents or delays the onset of any fibrosis or scarring within the tissues necessary for a normal erection. Now I think that a penile rehab program can start as early as a few weeks after the catheter is removed, especially once the man regains full urinary control (which will help him feel more confident in the bedroom and perform better sexually). Other methods like acupuncture may also be helpful; at this writing, studies on this are ongoing at our center.

So far, small studies show that penile rehabilitation improves a man's chances of restoring normal erectile function after surgery (as long as he has had nerve-sparing surgery and had normal erectile function *before* surgery). Speak with your doctor about penile rehabilitation if it's something you wish to pursue. Remember, if you don't use it, you could lose it!

Post-Prostatectomy Radiation

A large clinical study carried out by the Southwest Oncology Group (SWOG) has led us to believe that radiation will help men with high-risk disease—that is, cancer cells found in the margins, seminal vesicle involvement, or a Gleason score of 8 or more—to prevent a recurrence. Radiation given at this juncture is known as *adjuvant* radiation, which means it's given before any post-surgery rise in PSA. *(Salvage* radiation, on the other hand, is given after a post-surgery rise in PSA, and its benefits are less clear; see Chapter 7 for more on this.)

In the SWOG trial, radiation given following prostatectomy and before any rise in PSA post-surgery reduced the risk of biochemical (PSA) treatment failure by 50 percent over radical prostatectomy alone. Researchers tracked the PSA of 374 patients for an average of 10 years, starting immediately after prostate removal. Patients with a postsurgical PSA of 0.2 ng/ml who received radiation to the prostate bed after surgery were much less likely to have a recurrence. For patients with a postsurgical PSA between 0.2 and 1.0 ng/ml or higher, reductions in risk of biochemical failure, local failure, and distant failure were realized over the 10-year follow-up period.

From this large study, we can also deduce that treatment failure in high-risk patients is predominantly local. Most recurrences take place in the prostate bed (locally), and there is a surprisingly low incidence of distant (metastatic) failure. In other words, the best way to prevent distant treatment failure is to prevent local treatment failure. Adjuvant radiation to the prostate bed seems to reduce the risk of metastatic disease and biochemical failure postsurgery. Further improvement in reducing local treatment failure is likely to have the greatest impact on outcome in high-risk patients after prostatectomy.

Cryotherapy: Freezing Cancer to Death

With cryotherapy, just the area of the cancer is precisely targeted and killed (ablated) with one or more freezing needles. We do this by placing an ultrasound probe into the rectum to guide placement of several probes (cryoneedles) into cancerous areas of the prostate. Argon gas is then channeled through these needles to quickly cool and freeze cancerous areas. Once the tissue is frozen, argon or helium gas is run through the same needles to thaw the tissue.

Cryosurgery minimizes collateral tissue damage while effectively eradicating cancerous areas. This promising, low-risk therapy for localized prostate cancer is a particular area of expertise for me. I have performed cryosurgery on over 1,000 men and have taught it to urologists all over the world. You might hear this surgery referred to as cryosurgery, cryotherapy, cryoablation, or focal ablation.

At this writing, 7- to-8-year studies indicate that when cryosurgery is used as a primary treatment for localized or locally advanced disease (stages T1 to T3), it has a success rate of 89 to 92 percent. Cryosurgery is also used to treat patients who have had a cancer recurrence when radiation has failed, and we have had excellent long-term results with these patients: 97 percent of men treated survived for at least 10 years after the procedure.

When men are treated with radiation therapy only, 38 percent eventually have a recurrence, but only 12 percent of men have a positive biopsy following cryotherapy. Unlike prostatectomy, cryosurgery is effective for men whose cancers are likely to have grown just beyond the prostate or those who have aggressive (Gleason score at or above 7) tumors. It is also a good alternative for men who cannot have surgery or radiation or don't want to have either of these therapies. In the United States, the FDA has approved cryotherapy; Medicare covers it. In our experience, for patients who fail radiation therapy, the advantages of cryosurgery over radical prostatectomy are outstanding.

What to Expect from Cryotherapy

Some men who opt for "cryo" are advised to take medications that block the action of hormones on the prostate for a while before the procedure. This helps to shrink the gland, which makes the procedure easier to perform.

Currently, I recommend hormone ablation prior to cryotherapy to men whose prostate volume is over 60 grams. I suggest that these men take the hormones for 3 months before surgery. In addition to shrinking prostate size, these medications cause cancer cells to go into remission in most patients who take it under these circumstances. This is reflected in a drop in PSA—a drop that can sometimes range down into undetectable levels. If this happens to you, keep in mind that you still have cancer. Often, patients think that if they have a zero PSA on hormones, they no longer have cancer. This is untrue; it simply shows that hormone ablation therapy prevents cancer cells from making PSA. Some of the cells may die, but not all will die. Treatment with cryotherapy is still needed.

Modern-day cryosurgery is performed in the hospital or in

an outpatient center under either general or spinal (epidural) anesthesia. Most procedures take less than 90 minutes. No incision is made in this surgery. Because modern cryo uses pressurized argon gas instead of liquid nitrogen, the needles are extremely thin. This is about as minimally invasive as a surgery can get. We use ultrasound to guide the placement of the needles through the perineal region—the area of skin located under the scrotum. In two or more freeze-thaw cycles, we create "ice balls" that freeze cancer cells to a temperature where cell death occurs. Healthy tissues are protected from damage through a monitoring system: We insert probes called thermocouples and a urethral warming device to protect the urethra.

A urethral warmer is a catheter that is inserted before the freezing process. Warmed sterile water is pumped into the urethra, which prevents any damage there. In the days before we had the urethral warmer, complications involving urethral sloughing (where the man would painfully urinate dead urethral tissue for weeks or months), infection, and blockage of the urethra were common following cryosurgery. With today's excellent warming catheters, urethral sloughing occurs rarely, if ever.

Thermocouple devices introduced in the mid-1990s allow the surgeon to determine the extent of cell damage during the procedure and serve as an end point to the freezing cycle when temperatures below –40 degrees C are reached. Thermocouples also ensure that lethal temperatures are achieved in designated parts of the prostate and that adequately warm temperatures are maintained in surrounding areas.

One of the best features of this procedure is that there is no hospital stay—patients go home within a few hours after the procedure.

A small bandage is placed under the scrotum to protect the site where the needles were inserted while it heals. At Columbia University Medical Center in New York, we have performed over 1,000 of these procedures, and only one patient needed to stay overnight because of a slight fever. To date, not a single patient of mine has required a blood transfusion following cryo.

Cryoablation can cause some minor swelling of the prostate, which in theory could interfere with urine flow for a few days. To prevent this problem, we place a catheter in the bladder when we perform cryosurgery. Any swelling subsides within a few days, and we generally remove the catheter on the third day after the procedure.

How Cryosurgery Works

With the onset of ice formation, water is "extracted" from the outside of the cell walls. When this happens, water leaves the cell, followed by cell shrinkage. This is *cellular dehydration,* which causes damage. As the temperature falls to around –15 degrees C and below, ice starts to form inside the cell, which in turn causes the DNA of the cancer cells to break open and die.

Freezing also reduces the amount of oxygen available to cancer cells. Blood vessels in these areas freeze, leading to the rupture of tumor capillaries. Without blood flow through this capillary supply, cancer cells' oxygen levels drop, which further guarantees their demise.

The goal of the procedure is to kill all of the cells in the targeted area. The needles (also known as probes) can reach a uniform temperature of –40 degrees C in the tissue. We use software programs and transrectal ultrasound to determine the exact placement of the needles. Our aim is to ensure that every focus of cancer is eradicated. These tools enable us very accurately to place these needles while avoiding damage to adjacent structures.

Once the needles are placed, the surgeon sequentially freezes the prostate from the top of the gland (anterior) to the bottom of the gland (posterior). This sequencing supports clear visualization and control of the ice ball. Ice starts to grow at the tip of the needle and then grows backward on the needle a few centimeters. The amount of ice that is grown on the needle depends on how fast we flow the argon. For smaller prostates (less than 20 grams) we can grow the ice slower and generate smaller ice balls. If the prostate is large (over 40 grams), we can drive the argon much faster in the needles, giving us a larger ice ball to cover the tissue. The surgeon can watch the cancer being killed on the ultrasound monitor.

When we freeze a tissue with extreme cold, the result is called a cryolesion. If we look under the microscope at this lesion, we find dead cells in the center as well as an area around the center where cell death is apparent. In this procedure, cells that are closest to the cryoneedles will die first; the temperature there can drop as low as −80 degrees C! These cells quickly rupture as their cell walls break down. The cells farther from the tip die as the temperature reaches −40 degrees C. As we look outside these deeply frozen areas, the temperature gets warmer, and cells can remain alive. To ensure that we kill cancerous cells in the margins, not just at the center of the cryolesion, we place several needles for each cancerous area. The ice balls can then overlap to cover all margins.

Once temperatures have dropped adequately in the targeted

areas, the surgeon stops freezing and begins thawing. The thawing can be passive, where cells are allowed to warm up naturally, or active, where a warming gas is passed through the needles. Immediately post-thaw, some cancer cells will have experienced partial physical damage; they then undergo a process of cell death within an hour of thawing. Cells continue to die 6 to 12 hours after the procedure owing to biochemical stresses associated with the freeze.

Cryo works best when we use two cycles of freezing and thawing. Cancer cells stressed but not killed by the first bout of freezing are knocked out by the second bout. Damage to tumor blood supply allows us to cycle through the second freezing more rapidly and extends the area affected by the cold farther from the needles.

Cryosurgery Side Effects and Complications

Following cryosurgery, men may experience genital swelling and blood in the urine, but this lasts for only about a week. Earlier versions of this surgery led to high rates of fistula (where an opening was created between the urethra and the rectum); this is extremely rare today, occurring in less than 1 percent of patients. While urethral sloughing is also very rare with modern surgeries, it is more likely in men who have had transurethral resection of the prostate to treat prostate enlargement.

In the past, erectile dysfunction has been a major issue with cryosurgery, with rates as high as those for radical surgery. I believe this was because in the past, cryosurgeons were unable to measure the temperature along the nerve bundles, so the nerves were often damaged by the cooling/heating cycles. Early versions of this procedure involved ablating (freezing) the whole gland. Today, we have the ability to focus in on and freeze cancerous areas only, rather than freezing the entire prostate. This increased precision reduces the risk of postsurgery ED. Also, a temperature-monitoring system has been developed that allows surgeons to protect and spare erectile nerves. At this writing, a multicenter study of this monitoring system is under way.

Radiation Therapy

Although I did a bit of radiation bashing in an earlier chapter, the fact is that radiation can be very helpful for certain men with prostate cancer. Also known as radiotherapy, this treatment entails directing high-energy rays to damage cancer cells and thwart their growth. Radiotherapy affects cells only in the areas treated. It may be used:

- Instead of surgery or following surgery to get rid of any cancerous cells that have spread beyond the prostate

- In some high-risk patients who are not surgical candidates, in addition to hormonal therapy

- In patients with metastatic disease, to relieve pain or other problems caused when cancer has spread to the bones

We can administer radiotherapy either through direct beams of radiation from an external source (*external radiation*) or from a small capsule of radioactive material that is implanted directly into or near the tumor (*internal radiation*, also called brachytherapy). In some patients, we may use both internal and external radiation.

External radiation therapy is performed in an outpatient clinic. Doses of radiation are applied 5 days a week for about 7 to 9 weeks. Final treatments may include a radiation "boost" aimed at the area from which the tumor initially arose. X-rays and cobalt-60 gamma rays are two commonly used forms of radiation. You may also have the options of *intensity*-modulated *radiation therapy* (IMRT), *conformal radiation therapy*, or *proton beam therapy*. These forms of radiation are associated with less damage to surrounding normal tissues than older forms of radiation.

Intensity-modulated radiation therapy uses a CT scan to generate a three-dimensional picture of the prostate gland and surrounding organs, then targets the gland by means of thinner beams that are more precise than other forms of external beam radiation. We are thus able to administer a higher total dose of radiation to the gland while reducing exposures of surrounding tissues (rectum, bladder). IMRT is given 5 days a week over 7 to 8 weeks, in short sessions.

Conformal radiation therapy also uses computers to create a 3-D picture of the prostate, enabling radiation to be directed more precisely at the gland with less harm to surrounding healthy tissues. This enables us to use a higher dose to kill off cancer cells.

Proton beam radiation is an especially exciting development. We use 3-D technology to visualize the gland here as well, but protons are used to generate the radiation. Proton beams can pass through healthy tissues without damaging them yet can still be aimed at cancer tissue to destroy the cancerous cells. This type of therapy can precisely target the tumor while sparing surrounding tissues.

Proton beam radiation is believed to be associated with fewer side effects than older forms of radiation therapy, and it seems to be effective: In a recent study of proton beam therapy in 1,200 men with early-stage localized prostate cancer, 75 percent were disease-free 5 years later. If you are considering proton beam therapy, you should know that it will require at least 40 treatments over 2 months.

If you and your medical team decide on a radiation implant, expect a brief hospital stay for implantation. Just to be on the safe side, you will be cautioned to avoid close contact with others for a while following the placement of the implant (also known as a "seed"). The implant may be removed after a period of time, at which point it will no longer be radioactive; or it may be left in your body permanently. When the implant is left in, the treatment is referred to as brachytherapy.

The number of seeds implanted can vary depending on the size of the gland. Most radiation therapists prefer to do implantation only on men whose prostate volume is below 60 grams. In a gland larger than this, more seeds might have to be placed, which increases the risk of side effects like urinary retention and painful urination. If your prostate gland is over 60 grams, the radiation oncologist treating you is likely to suggest hormone therapy for at least 3 months, at which point he or she will repeat the prostate volume measurement with the aid of transrectal ultrasound. In rare cases, hormones will have to be continued for a longer period of time. As you'll find in a later section of this chapter, hormone ablation has its own side effects, including hot flashes, weight gain, and mood changes.

For the patient with low-risk features (PSA under 10 ng/ml and a Gleason score less than 7), most radiation oncologists administering brachytherapy will recommend the seed implant alone, without the external beam boost. Patients with intermediate or high-risk disease will likely be advised to have either the seed implant with external beam or external beam alone. With the external beam boost, oncologists can target a patient's seminal vesicles and lymph nodes as well as aiming beams at the tissues just beyond the prostate capsule, where seeds will not have a cancer-killing effect. For pain relief in patients with metastasized cancer, compounds like radioactive strontium can be injected directly into bone.

What about the men who were found to have positive nodes at the time of surgery? Does radiation help these men? Another study evaluated 1,921 patients who had prostate cancer treated with surgery alone or had surgery followed by radiation therapy. All of these patients had disease in the lymph nodes. No significant relative survival benefit was found for these men when they received postoperative radiation therapy. Data also do not support the routine use of radiation after surgery for men whose surgical specimens contain positive lymph nodes.

Radiation therapy can cure early-stage prostate cancer and can extend life even when cancer is advanced. Urinary symptoms and impotence are less common with radiation than with surgery, at least in the short term. Unfortunately, it's virtually impossible to avoid killing at least a few healthy cells around the area being targeted, no matter which form of radiation therapy you choose. Side effects are the result. During radiation therapy, you might experience:

- Fatigue

- Skin reactions in treated areas

- Frequent, painful urination

- Upset stomach

- Diarrhea

- Rectal bleeding or irritation

- Later development of impotence (in some patients who have external radiation)

- Decreased white blood cell and platelet counts (signs of decreased immune system function)

Radiation therapy also poses an added risk of secondary cancer development in the future. Several studies show that rates of rectal cancer and bladder cancer are increased following radiation to the pelvic area. If these cancers do develop, they tend to be rather aggressive, like those cancers in the prostate that recur after radiation. This is one of the reasons I am personally biased against radiation.

There's another reason I'm biased against radiation: In my practice, I see a lot of men who have already had radiation and failed. They are looking for an alternative, such as holistics or salvage cryotherapy.

If you do choose to undergo radiation therapy, seek out a major center that has treated thousands of patients.

Monitoring Treatment Success with PSA

After undergoing treatment, you'll have periodic PSA tests to monitor the success of those treatments. A rising PSA level after radiation or surgery usually suggests recurrent cancer. Urologists call this biochemical relapse, and it can occur without any clinical signs of cancer recurrence.

The definition of biochemical relapse following radical prostatectomy can vary from doctor to doctor. Most studies suggest that
a PSA value greater than 0.2 ng/ml after surgery is enough to
merit further treatment.

Following radiotherapy, PSA measurements can be less predictable, because the lowest PSA following treatment—also known
as the PSA nadir—isn't reached until 12 to 42 months after treatment ends. Most men who are considered cured have a PSA nadir
below 0.5 ng/ml, with no rise in PSA after that point.

In patients who have received radioactive implants, the PSA
may suddenly rise in the first 12 months after treatment. This phenomenon is referred to medically as a PSA bounce, and it's caused
by inflammation within the gland triggered by the treatment. PSA
values will go back down to nadir levels within a few months, and
no further therapy is required when a PSA bounce has occurred.

Not all rises in PSA following radiation are due to cancer. We
don't order a repeat prostate biopsy unless the patient has three
consecutive PSA rises. At that point, we routinely recommend a
biopsy to determine whether the rise is due to cancer. If further
testing reveals that cancer has spread, we begin to consider hormone therapy. If the cancer is still contained within the prostate
after radiation, I believe that salvage cryotherapy is an excellent
treatment choice.

High-intensity focused ultrasound (HIFU) is under investigation as a potential treatment for men with recurrence after
radiation. The preliminary data look promising for this form of
therapy, although at this writing it is not FDA-approved. Men
interested in HIFU will need to go outside the United States to
either Bermuda or Cancún, Mexico.

Refer to Chapter 7 for more information on rising PSA following radiation or surgical treatment.

Hormone Therapy for Prostate Cancer

Once prostate cancer has spread, or once it has recurred following surgery or radiation, your doctor may recommend hormone therapy, a mode of treatment based on our understanding of the growth-promoting effect of testosterone on prostate cancer. ("Hormone therapy" is a bit of a misnomer; here, it describes the use of drugs to *block* the action of hormones—with the exception of estrogens, which are actually hormones.) Hormone therapy involves the use of drugs that suppress or block the action of testosterone (to stop or slow the growth and spread of the cancer), and in rare cases it may include the use of estrogens to counteract the effects of testosterone in the body.

Hormone therapy isn't a cure, but it can stop disease progression in its tracks for 2 or more years. In 85 to 90 percent of men who start hormone therapy because of advanced prostate cancer, tumors shrink measurably. The problem is that cells within the prostate may become *hormone-refractory*—resistant to hormones—and these cells can continue to grow without the help of testosterone and eventually take over as the dominant cells in the cancer. At that point, hormone therapy can no longer keep the cancer at bay, and chemotherapy may be the only additional option for treatment.

Four classes of hormone drugs are used to treat prostate cancer:

1. Estrogens: These "female" hormones may counteract the effect of testosterone on prostate cancer cells. But because estrogen use increases the risk of heart attack, it is seldom prescribed today.

2. Luteinizing-hormone-releasing hormone (LHRH) agonists: These drugs block the effects of a hormone needed to trigger production of testosterone in the testicles. The drug creates a "chemical castration" that is less dire and more reversible than orchiectomy (surgical removal of the testicles, which was once a gold standard treatment for advanced prostate cancer). LHRH agonists do not address the testosterone produced in the adrenals, which are two walnut-sized glands that sit atop the kidneys. Five to 10 percent of a man's testosterone is produced there. Lupron, Trelstar, Vantas, Zoladex, and Viadur are LHRH agonists, and all but Viadur are given by injection every 1 to 4 months (Viadur is given as a once-a-year implant in the arm). LHRH agonists can cause side effects that include the disappearance of sex drive, hot flashes, gynecomastia (breast growth) or painful breasts, fatigue, muscle loss, weight gain, and lowered levels of "good" HDL cholesterol.

When LHRH agonists are first administered, they can cause an initial *tumor flare*—an acceleration of the cancer's growth. The prostate may become enlarged, and bladder obstruction can result. For men with bone metastases, this flare can cause major problems, including bone pain, fractures, and nerve compression. Giving antiandrogens (described below) first and then switching to LHRH agonists after the initial period can help men to reduce or avoid tumor flare.

3. Antiandrogens: These drugs work at the cellular level to block the effects of testosterone on prostate cancer cells. Overall, side effects are not as severe with antiandrogens because they don't prevent testosterone production. These medications are given as daily pills. Potential side effects include breast tenderness, nausea, and diarrhea, but their effect on libido is less severe than with LHRH agonists. Interestingly, if antiandrogens don't work to slow cancer growth, stopping the drug may slow the cancer down. Sometimes LHRH agonists and antiandrogens are used together. Some urological oncologists are experimenting with intermittent hormone therapy, where hormone blockade is given in a discontinuous way so that the body can have breaks from side effects. At this writing, research on this is promising—it suggests that intermittent therapy works just as well as consistent use of these medicines.

4. LHRH antagonists: This is the newest class of hormone-ablating medications; it received FDA approval while I wrote this book. LHRH antagonists affect receptor sites in the brain, causing them to stop releasing a hormone needed for testosterone production in the testicles. Given as a monthly injection, this drug—called degarelix (brand name Firmagon, from Ferring Pharmaceuticals)—is injected into the fat underneath the skin of the belly once a month. It results in a very rapid reduction in blood testosterone levels. With degarelix, there is no flare phenomenon, so no antiandrogen is needed during treatment.

In a recent study that compared Lupron with degarelix, men in the degarelix group did better: They maintained lower levels of testosterone and better PSA-relapse-free survival. Both groups experienced hot flashes and impotence, which is not surprising since the medicine seriously lowers testosterone levels.

My personal feeling is that the flare phenomenon is an important consideration in high-risk patients, including men with metastatic disease or those with rapidly rising PSA. If you experience a PSA relapse after surgery or radiation, and there is no disease on a bone or CT scan, it may not make that much difference whether you use degarelix or Lupron. At this writing, Lupron can be administered only once every 3 months, while degarelix is available only as a 1-month treatment. If you'd rather not have to see your urologist every month, Lupron would be the winner.

PSA and Hormonal Therapy

The ideal PSA value for men on hormones is less than 0.1 ng/ml, which would indicate that the cancer is not biologically active. It is important for patients and physicians to understand, as I mentioned previously, that a zero PSA on hormones does not necessarily mean that the patient is cancer-free. Hormones shut off the ability of the cancer cell to make PSA, but it is not a cure—the patient may still have cancer.

Many aggressive cancer cells can make less PSA or no PSA at all. We need to ensure that men on hormone ablation therapy periodically have other tests performed to measure cancer activity, such as bone scans and CT scans of the pelvis. It isn't possible to predict how long PSA will stay low on hormones; this number varies based on the extent of cancer and the biological nature of the cells within the tumor.

Hormone-Refractory Prostate Cancer: Next Steps

If PSA starts to rise when a patient is on hormones, this is a reflection of uncontrolled disease. The cancer has developed resistance and is no longer under hormonal control. This form of prostate cancer is referred to as androgen-insensitive, hormone-refractory, or castrate-resistant. These patients should seek advice from a medical oncologist about the role of other medications, such as antiandrogens, antifungals (Nizoral), or chemotherapy, to bring the cancer back under control.

The newest form of treatment for these patients has been *immunotherapy*. A drug called Provenge has received approval by the FDA for use in men with minimal disease in the bone and a rising PSA. Provenge can improve survival in men with late-stage cancers, and overall it is well tolerated. The most common side affects are chills, nausea, fever, and joint pains.

This form of therapy relies on your body's own immune system to fight cancer. Patients can expect to receive a total of three infusions every 2 weeks, where some of his own white cells are removed and exposed to a prostate-specific protein called prostate acid phosphatase. Those "charged" cells are then reinfused back into the patient's body.

In the study supporting use of this treatment, men who received immunotherapy lived, on average, 4 months longer than men in the placebo group of the study. I know that probably doesn't sound all that great, but many men in the study lived much longer than expected; these were men who already had advanced disease. The therapy is not cheap, however. At this writing, the cost is nearly $90,000. Most oncologists, myself included, aren't sure how insurance companies are going to pay for this. It may be a therapy that will ultimately be accessible only to the very wealthy.

CHAPTER 7

RISING PSA AFTER TREATMENT

Every week, I see around 10 patients who have already run the gauntlet of prostate cancer treatment . . . and now their PSA is rising again. They want to know what to do.

This is a common scenario. According to statistics drawn from a large Medicare database, 25 to 50 percent of men who have had some form of definitive therapy such as surgery or radiation will have a rising PSA in the aftermath. These men show up in my office wanting to know, "Why is my PSA rising? Is this rise worrisome? Is it cancer? Do I need more treatment?"

Remember: The PSA test is not a cancer test. When PSA rises in a man undergoing initial screening, it can indicate the presence of cancer, but it doesn't have to. But how about the man who has already had cancer surgery? What about radiation therapy?

In this chapter, I'll tell you how we respond to these patients: what tests we use to figure out why PSA is rising again, how we determine whether more treatment is called for, and what benefits and risks you are likely to encounter if you undergo these treatments.

As you read, keep in mind that the decision-making process when PSA rises following treatment is rarely an easy one. It's not often a "red light/green light" situation where the way forward is clear and simple; expect lots of yellow lights and yield signs here. Hard choices might present themselves, physician opinions on what's best might differ, and research studies haven't yet given us enough information to create an algorithm that works in each case of rising PSA following treatment. Ultimately, our goal is to catch any recurrence while it is still local, in the bed of the prostate or near it, so that it doesn't turn into distant (metastasized) disease.

Our course of action depends upon the treatments the man has already had: We'll take one course with a man who has had a radical prostatectomy and a different course with a man who has undergone radiation therapy, cryosurgery, or high-intensity focused ultrasound (HIFU), for example.

Post-treatment, a few different outcomes are possible:

1. PSA will remain low and you'll never have a recurrence.
2. *Biochemical failure*, where PSA rises again but there is no visible evidence of cancer on CT scan, bone scan, or any imaging. This is common—it happens in up to 30 percent of men who have had their prostates removed.
3. *Local failure*, where PSA rises as disease recurs in the area of the prostate.
4. *Distant failure*, where PSA rises as metastases show up in parts of the body distant to the prostate—lymph nodes, bone, or (rarely) soft tissues like liver and lung.

To determine which of these four outcomes might be responsible for a rise in PSA, we go through a fairly complex process of diagnostic deduction. Ultimately, our goal is to try to catch a recurrence of prostate cancer while it is still local—in the area of the prostate gland, seminal vesicles and surrounding lymph nodes.

Whether the gland has been removed or not, we will have a better chance of successfully treating a recurrence when it's local.

Rising PSA after Surgery

When a man comes to me after radical prostatectomy with a report of a rising PSA and no other complaints, the first thing I look at is the pathology report from the surgery. I want to know whether cancer was found in the margins, seminal vesicles, or lymph nodes.

If cancer was found outside the prostate, the man clearly has a higher risk of PSA relapse, because prostate cancer cells anywhere in the body will make PSA. In these men, a rising PSA would suggest that the cancer has begun to grow and spread. Among men believed to be "cured" by radical prostatectomy, about 10 percent see their PSA rise to a level that indicates a cancer recurrence after surgery (PSA over 0.2 ng/ml).

If no cancer was found outside of the prostate, how can PSA rise once the gland is removed? One possibility is that non-cancerous prostate tissue was left at the bladder neck at the time of surgery. This can happen even in the hands of an expert robotic surgeon, especially in men who have a large median lobe (prostate tissue growing up into the bladder). Even benign bladder neck tissue will create enough PSA to be detectable with the tests we use following surgery. If transrectal ultrasound reveals a mass of tissue at the *anastomosis* (where the urethra was reconnected to the bladder), it should be biopsied; if it turns out to be benign, I usually recommend a course of Avodart. This tends to reduce the PSA within 3 months, and no further treatment is likely to be needed.

If this doesn't explain a rising PSA following surgery, we then look at 1) the timing of the PSA rise following surgery; and 2) whether the PSA ever went to undetectable levels.

PSA should be less than 0.1 ng/ml at 6 weeks following treatment. If PSA is higher than this at that point, some prostate cells have likely been left behind. They may be benign, but more often they turn out to be cancerous. Under these circumstances, it's important to look carefully at the pathology result to see where the PSA-producing cells are coming from.

If one or more lymph nodes were positive or if the seminal vesicles were involved, the PSA-producing cells may be systemic; hormone therapy is the usual next measure. Studies show that in men with positive lymph nodes after surgery, hormone ablation improves survival and prevents bone metastasis. Although salvage radiation may be recommended for these men with persistently elevated PSA, the role of that treatment is unclear. (*Salvage* denotes that the radiation is given when PSA has started to rise; *adjuvant* radiation denotes radiation therapy given in the absence of a rise in PSA.) So far, it appears that radiation given at this juncture may not impact survival or extend periods free of disease.

As you learned in Chapter 6, some patients start out with undetectable PSA 6 weeks following surgery even if pathology reports reveal positive margins (cancer just outside the prostate) or seminal vesicle involvement. These men are considered at high risk for disease relapse, which usually manifests first as a PSA elevation. Giving them adjuvant radiation after surgery and before rise in PSA after surgery seems to improve their chances of a cure.

Post-Surgery Radiation in Men with Biochemical (PSA) Relapse

So-called *salvage* radiation is performed in some cases where post-surgery PSA is slowly rising. Research hasn't yet revealed any hard-and-fast cutoff point where salvage radiation should begin, but in my clinical experience, it's best to do it before PSA goes past 1.0. If PSA has already relapsed to 2.0 or more, it's too late to try to do radiation.

If you've been told that any PSA relapse calls for radiation, keep in mind that this issue is still controversial. PSA relapse (biochemical recurrence) after radical prostatectomy does not always mean systemic progression or that the man will die from prostate cancer. Approximately one-third of patients with biochemical failure will have only local recurrence.

This was borne out in a study, published in 2011, that evaluated 14,632 patients who underwent surgery at the Mayo Clinic between 1990 and 2006. Of these, 2,426 men were found to have a recurrence, defined by a PSA level of 0.4 ng/ml or higher. None of them had any radiation after surgery, and they were tracked for an average of 11.5 years. Here's how the figures played out with regard to death from cancer during this period, relative to the length of time following surgery that the PSA relapse occurred:

- Of men who experienced relapse less than 1.2 years postsurgery, just over 90 percent were alive at the end of follow-up.

- Of men who experienced relapse 1.2 to 3.1 years postsurgery, 90.7 percent were alive at the end of follow-up.

- Of men who experienced relapse 3.1 to 5.9 years postsurgery, 92.2 percent were alive at the end of follow-up.

- Of men who experienced relapse more than 5.9 years postsurgery, 95.3 percent were alive at the end of follow-up.

Overall, the results of this study strongly suggest that only a minority of men experience systemic progression and death from prostate cancer following a PSA relapse. Because the benefit of initial adjuvant radiation treatment is unclear here, the decision to start a secondary therapy such as radiation must balance out the risk of the morbidity of treatment. Some men choose to forego radiation under these circumstances, and instead begin an intensive holistic program in conjunction with ongoing monitoring.

The timing of the PSA relapse after surgery is also important. Men whose PSA was undetectable for more than a year and then rises are likely experiencing a different situation from those who have a rise in the first few months. Men with a local recurrence probably won't see PSA jump until years after surgery; in men with metastatic disease, PSA will tend to spike early on after surgery.

Other studies have looked at the relationship between PSA doubling time and risk of death from prostate cancer following treatment. Those studies suggest that a man whose PSA doubling time is longer than 6 months has a better prognosis than a man with a shorter doubling time. In my experience, men with short PSA doubling times (6 months or less) don't benefit from radiation therapy; they benefit most from hormone ablation. These men don't have to use hormones for life, but at least 7 months of therapy are often required to bring PSA down to undetectable levels and achieve a biochemical remission, where prostate cancer cells no longer produce PSA. This doesn't mean the patient is cancer-free, but that his cancer is no longer active. Patients who go this route may then be able to start intermittent hormone deprivation (a "holiday" period during which hormones are not used).

PSA Rise after Radiation

As discussed in a previous chapter, radiation is a common form of therapy for patients with newly diagnosed, localized prostate cancer. Nearly a third of newly diagnosed prostate cancer patients will choose one form of radiation therapy as their primary treatment. Despite modifications in the ways we deliver radiation to the gland (including intensity modulation, 3-D conformal, and computer-assisted seed implantation), a significant number of these patients will see their PSA rise during the years following radiation.

It's tough to know what course of action to take in this situation. Urologists have not been well educated about how best to manage these men. For most, the knee-jerk reaction to a rising PSA after radiation is to start men on hormone therapy without doing an evaluation. I'll say it again: Not all PSA rises after treatment are due to cancer—and that includes PSA rises after radiation therapy.

Patients often ask me why radiation did not eradicate their prostate cancer. One possibility is that the radiation dose wasn't high enough to get rid of all cancer cells. We now know that radiation dose is a key component of whether or not a patient will have a PSA relapse after treatment. The higher the dose, the more likely it is the patient will become cancer-free.

So why don't we give the highest dose we can? Because higher doses are typically associated with more side effects—specifically, damage to the rectum, urethra, and bladder. Higher radiation doses are also more likely to cause erectile dysfunction and urinary incontinence, and they carry a greater chance of spurring the formation of a secondary malignancy (bladder and rectal cancers can occur years later in men treated with pelvic and prostate radiation). So radiation therapy can fail if we don't administer the dose that will get rid of all cancer cells.

Remember that all prostate cancer cells make PSA, whether they are in the prostate or have metastasized to another part of the body; and PSA elevation doesn't have to mean cancer at all. These factors make it difficult to clearly define whether a man needs additional local treatment (cryosurgery, HIFU), systemic treatment via hormone ablation, or no treatment at all.

Evaluating the Patient
Whose PSA Rises Post-Radiation

If the PSA should rise in a patient who has already undergone radiation therapy, the optimal time for intervention is unclear. Most radiation oncologists feel that PSA fluctuation within the first few years is not necessarily a problem that has to be addressed right away; in fact, a temporary PSA rise after brachytherapy is commonly seen around 20 months following treatment. Some evidence suggests that when this "PSA bounce" phenomenon is seen in patients following a seed implant, it may portend a poorer outcome, but this has not been conclusively established. I have seen many patients with PSA bounce, and in my experience the majority have a PSA elevation because of inflammation; in treating these patients, I have used an herbal approach (see following) that has been very successful.

At this writing, there is no consensus among urologists or radiation oncologists as to whether treatment should be given when PSA rises after radiation. When considering salvage therapy, the clinician needs to take into account other variables such as preexisting medical conditions, age of the patient, and patient preference. In my practice, I consider a biopsy a reasonable step if PSA rises above the lowest level three times in a row.

Under these circumstances, a biopsy should retrieve multiple cores—12 or more. When PSA rises post-radiation, I also recommend a biopsy of the seminal vesicles on each side, because the likelihood of seminal vesicle involvement in men with locally recurrent disease is fairly high. If seminal vesicle involvement is found, hormone therapy might be indicated along with additional local therapy.

If a prostate biopsy reveals recurrent disease in the gland, I generally suggest performing a metastatic evaluation—including a CT scan of the abdomen and pelvis and a bone scan. In high-risk patients, an open or laparoscopic biopsy of the pelvic lymph nodes might be called for, although for the most part I have stopped performing this test. Surgical removal of the nodes in a man who has had radiation is not easy and can cause significant side effects.

A few modern imaging tests like the capromab pendetide (CP) test (Cytogen Corporation, Princeton, New Jersey) may come in handy here. The CP test radioactively tags a specific antibody, then uses a scan to identify places where that antibody is active. This shows us where cancer may have spread.

The CP test helps us spare patients the undue morbidity of local salvage procedures (which won't do much good in the man whose cancer has spread—we'd likely turn to hormone ablation in those cases) and offers us an opportunity for cure in selected high-risk patients whose disease is still local. In those men, we can also avoid premature use of hormone therapy.

Other Factors and Modes of Salvage Therapy

At this writing, urologists don't have complete guidelines to follow in selecting patients for *salvage therapy*—a blanket term for a medical therapy used after initial treatments fail. In the United States, current salvage therapies for prostate cancer recurrence include salvage cryoablation, radical surgery, brachytherapy, and high-intensity focused ultrasound. Optimal candidates for these procedures would be those with evidence of locally recurrent disease and without evidence of metastatic disease, PSA less than 10 ng/ml, PSA doubling time longer than 6 months, no evidence of seminal vesicle invasion, and a life expectancy greater than 10 years.

I have extensive experience with cryoablation therapy in the salvage setting, and I have to come clean here: I have a bias toward this procedure based on my patients' positive experience with it. See Chapter 6 for the full story on cryoablation. The long-term outcome for the patients I treat is excellent: At 10 years, over 90 percent of these men are disease-free, and I have been able to spare many from hormone therapy after cryosurgery. Moreover, if cancer should return after salvage cryotherapy, it is possible to have a second cryotherapy; this is not the case with radiation.

At Columbia, we followed up with 76 men who had either

post-radiation cryosurgery (51 patients) or primary cryosurgery (25 patients) 10 or more years earlier. The average age of these men was just over 69 years; their PSA measurements ranged from 0.2 ng/ml to 208 ng/ml before cryosurgery; and their average Gleason score was 7. Seven of the men had high-risk disease. After 10 years of follow-up, 43 (55 percent) of the 76 men were still alive; 33 men (43.4 percent) had died, but only 10 of them (13.2 percent) from prostate cancer.

Some would say that the best tactic with local recurrence of prostate cancer following radiation is a salvage radical prostatectomy. I've participated in debates about this at national conferences. To date, I haven't seen any reason why a man who has undergone radiation for prostate cancer and who then has a local recurrence should undergo a salvage radical prostatectomy. I have reviewed the data and there is *no difference* in overall survival between men who have had radical surgery and those who have had cryosurgery.

There is, however, a big difference in terms of negative postprocedure side effects. Almost half of the men who have their prostates removed end up wearing diapers; less than 5 percent of cryosurgery patients do. Rates of rectal injury are much higher in men who have salvage prostatectomy than in men who have cryoablation, even when the surgery is performed by someone expert in the former procedure. Salvage prostatectomy is a very difficult operation; only a handful of doctors should even attempt it.

Few doctors offer salvage radiation to men who have already failed radiation. Some radiation doctors believe that perhaps the initial dose was too low and that by boosting the dose through the placement of radioactive seeds, they might achieve a more successful outcome. It never made a lot of sense to me to give a man more radiation when it has already failed, and I would be nervous about long-term side effects in men who get a double dose of this form of therapy.

High-intensity focused ultrasound is one of the newest treatments available for men with recurrent cancer after radiation. (HIFU is used for primary treatment, too; see page 117 for a review.) Not surprisingly, complications in patients after salvage HIFU are much more likely than after primary HIFU.

Urinary incontinence is the most frequent complication after salvage HIFU. Studies show that 20 to 50 percent of patients experience leakage of urine following this procedure. In some of these men, leakage can be severe enough to require an artificial urinary sphincter implantation. Rectourethral fistula (where a hole is opened up between the rectum and the urethra) is a rare complication after salvage HIFU. Side effects like these are more common in salvage HIFU than in primary HIFU—not surprising, considering that tissue that has already been irradiated may be less viable and have poor blood supply. HIFU is not currently FDA-approved for salvage therapy, but the treatment is currently undergoing clinical trials around the country.

What about Holistic Treatments?

Many men with a slow-rising PSA after radiation and surgery can manage their disease with active holistic surveillance. If there is concern about cancer after radiation, a prostate biopsy should be done; but what if there is no cancer on the biopsy and the scans are clean?

How about the man with a biopsy that shows just a small amount of cancer? I have successfully helped many men in these situations opt for active holistic surveillance without salvage treatments.

As you already know if you've read this far, diet and lifestyle can have a significant impact on cancer progression. By implementing the diet, supplement, and lifestyle modification plans in this book, you may be able to control PSA and cancer without having to accept the hazards inherent in Western medicine.

Follow the guidelines given for the chemoprevention diet and supplements in chapters 8 and 9. In particular, avoid red meat, dairy (aside from yogurt), fried foods, and sugars and eat more fresh vegetables. Drink 3 cups of green tea a day and exercise four to five times a week. When cooking oil is called for, use olive oil and avoid polyunsaturated vegetable oils like corn oil and soybean oil.

Take the following supplements (some of these are recommended in Chapter 9 for chemoprevention):

- The mushroom supplement active hexose correlated compound (AHCC), two pills twice a day (Quality of Life Labs: 877-937-2422 or http://www.q-o-l.com)

- Genistein concentrated polysaccharide (GCP), which is made from fermented soy, two pills twice a day

- Broccoli supplement BroccoProtect, three pills a day (Designs for Health: 800-367-4325 or http://www.designsforhealth.com)

- Vitamin D3, 5,000 IU a day (I suggest getting a baseline vitamin D level at the start of active holistic surveillance after treatment)

- Zyflamend from New Chapter, three pills a day

- Fish oil, two pills a day

- LycoPom from New Chapter, two capsules a day

- Daily men's vitamin: Every Man by New Chapter

Be sure you have a baseline PSA when starting active holistic surveillance and have another PSA test every 3 months for the next 2 years while on the protocol. Have the PSA measured in the same lab each time to ensure consistency.

PART III

CHEMOPREVENTION, YOUR PROSTATE, AND YOUR HEALTH

CHAPTER 8

THE PROSTATE CANCER DIET

Whether a man's prostate cancer is advanced or fast-growing enough to require allopathic treatments or he is advised to watch and wait, he can do a lot to support his body's ability to vanquish the disease and boost the functioning of his immune system. The same is true for men who have already undergone treatment and wish to do all they can to avoid a recurrence. At the Center for Holistic Urology at Columbia University Medical Center, we are constantly evolving in our recommendations to men who are open to a program of diet changes, nutritional supplements, stress relief, and exercise. This program, when combined with careful monitoring, is what we call active holistic surveillance.

We incorporate a broad range of natural therapies in prostate cancer treatment plans, including foods like pomegranate, cruciferous vegetables, flaxseeds, and soy and herbs like turmeric, ginger, oregano, rosemary, garlic, and green tea. In this chapter, you'll learn how specific foods, herbs, and nutrients prevent, slow, or even reverse unwanted changes in the prostate and how the wrong foods may impact prostate health and make cancer more likely to develop, grow, and spread.

Nutrition's Role in Prostate Cancer

African American men have the highest risk of prostate cancer on the planet: These men are *60 times* more likely to develop prostate cancer than men who are at lowest risk (those who live in Shanghai, China). White American men have a 43-fold greater risk than men from Shanghai. Canadian men, Swedish men, Australian men, and French men have a 20-fold or greater likelihood of receiving a prostate cancer diagnosis compared with those lucky guys from Shanghai. Middle-of-the-road risk is found in Denmark, the United Kingdom, Italy, Spain, and Israel. And Asian nations—Singapore, Japan, Hong Kong, India, and China—have the lowest risk.

Does this mean that something about being Asian is protective? This seems like a logical conclusion until we look at the way risk shifts in men who move from low-risk to high-risk countries. Data on the Pakistani and Indian immigrant population in the United States, for example, found that while the top male cancer in India is oral cancer, the risk of prostate cancer in Indian men in the United States is comparable to that of native-born American men. When a man adopts the lifestyle and diet of a high-risk country, his risk rises correspondingly. These changes in risk are linked to changes in diet and lifestyle that most immigrants adopt when they make the United States their home. These men exercise less and eat a diet heavier in fats, alcohol, and meat and lower in fiber. When in Rome, do as the Romans do; when in America, eat and exercise as the Americans do—and be rewarded with a higher risk of prostate cancer!

As more of the planet eats like Americans, the incidence of prostate cancer is rising even in relatively low-risk countries. This further supports the notion that diet plays a strong role in prostate cancer risk. Just how does diet impact a man's prostate gland in ways that predispose him to developing cancer there? Good question—and it's one to which we're slowly finding answers through nutritional research.

To understand how what goes into a man's mouth might impact his prostate, we do several different kinds of studies. First, we might look at the diets of different groups of people and track their incidence of prostate cancer in order to determine what dietary habits seem most strongly correlated with higher or lower risk. We can then hone in on the most likely causal factors and do more precise research on those factors.

For example, there is considerable evidence across populations that men who eat more meat (in particular meat that has been charred, creating *poly-aromatic hydrocarbons*) and more full-fat dairy products have a higher risk of prostate cancer. We also know that men who eat diets with more vegetables, herbs (especially Asian herbs like turmeric and ginger), and green tea have a much lower risk. Once we start to see these kinds of relationships between behaviors and risk, we can do test-tube and animal experiments using prostate cancer cell lines and animals that have had prostate cancer cells implanted into their bodies. We can expose those cells to compounds found in meat and dairy to see what kind of carcinogenic mechanisms are at play, and to compounds abundant in vegetables and green tea to see how these foods are protective. We can study the impact of these compounds at different stages of carcinogenesis and cancer progression.

Overall, these kinds of studies paint a big picture of the ways in which foods and the compounds they contain impact cells' likelihood of shifting from healthy to cancerous (that's carcinogenesis) and of becoming more aggressive and likely to spread (that's progression and metastasis). Here's what that picture looks like, in broad strokes.

Dietary Factors and Prostate Cancer: The Big Picture

The foods we eat deliver needed *macronutrients* like carbohydrates, proteins, and fats. Macronutrients are our sources of *calories*, or energy that powers the cellular "engines" that keep us alive and functioning. Food is also the source of *micronutrients* like vitamins, minerals, and *phytochemicals* (plant chemicals) that play multiple roles in every aspect of the body's function at the cellular level. Our bodies can't produce any of these nutrients on their own; we need to take them in every day through the food we eat.

All food is not created equal. Whole, natural foods and processed junk foods both contain macronutrients and micronutrients, yes. But the nutritional content of whole, natural foods is quite different from that of processed junk both in *nutrient density* (the amount of vitamins, minerals, and phytochemicals per calorie) and in its content of potentially harmful compounds like refined sugars, poly-aromatic hydrocarbons, unhealthy fats, and added hormones, pesticides, and other chemicals often used in the processed food industry.

To review: Some foods are especially full of health-promoting micronutrients, while others are especially full of harmful compounds. Certain foods—in particular some of the herbs I'll recommend in the next chapter as supplements—pack a supersized nutritional punch. They are very dense in the nutrients most likely to help promote better health and reduce cancer risk. And some of these "superfoods" contain novel healing compounds that are not found in most of the foods we normally eat.

When we supplement the body with herbs or micronutrients, we're trying to harness the power of those health-promoting nutrients to counteract the imbalances that lead to cancer growth. In body cells—including the cells of the prostate gland—this fight of good foods versus not-so-good foods impacts the balance of two processes that can make or break the body's resistance to cancer development or progression. Working with nutrition to modulate the balance of these interrelated processes is at the heart of holistic oncology.

Chronic inflammation/immune system balance

As you learned on pages 28 to 29, inflammation is the immune system's way of targeting and eliminating pathogens (bacteria, viruses) and initiating the healing process following injury. It involves the migration of immune cells to wherever they're needed and their action once they arrive. These specialized cells are designed to fight off unwanted invaders and draw the body's healing resources to the area. This is *acute* inflammation. We don't want to prevent it, as the body could not heal without it.

Chronic inflammation is the subject of concern here. When inflammation becomes chronic, the immune system never quite seems to get the message to cease and desist. Cells in the area of inflammation become chronically irritated by the action of the immune system. And while this chronic, low-grade inflammation may not play a role in initiating cancer, it does seem to help cancer formation in cells that have already made genetic shifts that predispose them to cancer—a state called dysplasia.

We've known for some time that certain cancers have a link to long-term, slow-burning infections or irritations that create a chronic state of inflammation. Cervical cancer has a link with human papillomavirus infection; stomach cancer, with infection by *Helicobacter pylori* bacteria; irritants in cigarette smoke cause chronic inflammation in the airways and mouth, predisposing the smoker to lung or mouth cancer; chronic irritation of the esophagus due to gastroesophageal reflux raises the risk of esophageal cancer.

Bladder cancer can also spring from chronic inflammation. One of the most aggressive forms of bladder cancer that I have treated in my career, squamous cell carcinoma, is found only in men and women with a history of multiple urinary tract infections. In Egypt, the most common form of bladder cancer develops through a parasitic infection called schistosomiasis, which is caused by parasites that attach to the skin, penetrate it, and migrate through the venous system to the bladder, where the parasites lay their eggs. Over time, the eggs cause an intense chronic inflammation that often leads to cancer development.

It appears that other cancers have a less obvious but no less real link to slow-burning inflammation—prostate cancer included. This link was first suspected when researchers found that men who had a history of prostatitis (prostate inflammation) or sexually transmitted infections had a higher risk of developing prostate cancer. Long-term use of anti-inflammatory drugs (described on page 47) and diets high in antioxidants (which help counter inflammation) have been linked with lower risk. Even before the development of PIN, pro-inflammatory atrophy can be seen in areas that eventually become PIN and prostate cancer. In multiple studies where cancerous and non-cancerous prostate tissues are carefully examined and their biochemical activities studied, a clear relationship has emerged between inflammation and the formation, growth, and spread of prostate cancer.

In 2006, researchers discovered a new virus in patients with prostate cancer—XMRV, which is a close relative of a virus associated with leukemia. Since that discovery, several studies have examined the possible relationship between XMRV and prostate cancer. None provided substantial evidence that this virus causes prostate cancer.

Inflammation that doesn't shut itself off has been implicated as a factor in many health problems aside from cancer. We've long known that so-called autoimmune diseases like rheumatoid arthritis, lupus, some kinds of thyroid disease, and Crohn's disease are caused by an immune system that seems to have lost its natural controls. Just since the 1990s, investigations into links between chronic inflammation and heart disease, depression, stroke, adult-onset diabetes, and Alzheimer's disease have gathered a lot of momentum. It follows that by adopting an anti-inflammatory program of chemoprevention, you'll enjoy benefits that reach well beyond your prostate gland.

Although our bodies' propensity toward chronic inflammation is in part genetically determined, the foods we eat have an impact on how that genetic blueprint plays out. Inflammation is mediated by hormonelike chemicals called eicosanoids (eye-KAH-suh-noyds). Some eicosanoids encourage chronic inflammation; others discourage it. They impact the action of the immune system as well as the constriction of blood vessels, blood clotting, stomach acid secretion, and the intensity and longevity of pain and fever. And eicosanoids are built from polyunsaturated fats in the foods we eat. The fats we consume dictate the action of enzymes that build eicosanoids. Certain enzymes make "good," anti-inflammatory eicosanoids; others make "bad," pro-inflammatory eicosanoids.

"Good" eicosanoids are made from omega-3 fats, which are found in fish, walnuts, flaxseeds, and leafy green vegetables. "Bad" eicosanoids are made from omega-6 fats, found in most of the vegetable oils used to make processed foods, including oils made from corn, soybeans, sunflower, safflower, and cottonseed. Meats and dairy products, which come mostly from animals that are fed a grain-rich diet, also are high in omega-6s. The body's production of eicosanoids depends in large part on the balance of these fats in the diet. Add to this the fact that refined carbohydrates (bread, pastry, pasta, crackers, sugary treats) affect the biochemical process that produces eicosanoids, encouraging the production of more of the "bad" (pro-inflammatory) variety, and you can see why Americans tend to be way out of balance when it comes to eicosanoids and inflammation. In a body that's predisposed to excess chronic inflammation because of poor diet, cancer may be better able to gain purchase and grow more quickly.

Dozens of eicosanoids are made in the human body. In prostate cancer, the eicosanoid-building enzymes that seem to have the greatest impact on progression are *cyclooxygenase-2* (COX-2), *5-lipoxygenase* (5-LOX), and *12-lipoxygenase* (12-LOX). These enzymes lead to the production of pro-inflammatory eicosanoids like *prostaglandin E2* and *leukotriene B4*. In the next chapter, you will learn about how herbs can be used to gently modulate these enzymes in ways that help to explain their beneficial effects on prostate cancer and PIN.

Allopathic medicine treats chronic inflammation with drugs that impact eicosanoid production and action by altering the balance of these and other enzymes. Steroid drugs like prednisone do this very efficiently, but their side effects are extreme, making them worth using only when a patient's survival or mobility is at stake (for example, in severe cases of autoimmune disease). NSAIDs such as aspirin, ibuprofen, and naproxen are more commonly used to control inflammation. NSAIDs do reduce inflammation, but large-scale studies haven't consistently demonstrated that they help to prevent cancer unless they are taken for many years on a regular basis.

Besides, there are risks with NSAIDs that make them an unacceptable preventive measure. Gastrointestinal bleeding is a common issue with long-term use of these medications, because they impact the stomach's ability to protect itself against the acids it makes to digest food. The COX-2 inhibitor drugs developed to try to avoid gastrointestinal bleeding as a side effect turned out to dramatically raise the risk of heart problems and strokes, so they can't be used long-term. (COX-2 drugs are being used to try to prevent cancer in a very specific population: those who have large numbers of colon polyps that are likely to turn cancerous.)

NSAIDs have highly targeted actions that interrupt only part of the inflammation process. COX-2 inhibitors target the production of only one eicosanoid-forming enzyme; older-guard NSAIDs block both COX-2 and another enzyme called COX-1. COX-1 isn't a major player in inflammation, but when we block it along with COX-2, we disrupt the balance of these two enzymes in a way that impacts the production of acids in the stomach. This is why old-guard NSAIDs increase risk of intestinal bleeding, and why drug researchers believed that blocking only COX-2 would give us better anti-inflammatory effect without the risk of bleeding. Unfortunately, we found that in increasing the drug's specificity, we created another, even less desirable side effect: a drastic increase in risk of heart attacks and strokes.

In holistic medicine, there is a belief that if you disrupt only one small aspect of a physiological process with a drug—which is, after all, what most drugs are designed to do—you throw the whole system into imbalance. Anti-inflammatory diet shifts and herbal medicines modulate inflammation more gently.

Oxidant/antioxidant balance

Cells metabolize—"burn"—food as fuel. Into the cell go carbohydrates, fats, or proteins, and as this fuel is burned, energy is released from the cells. Also released is a kind of cellular "exhaust" made up of unpaired electrons, otherwise known as free radicals. Electrons prefer to travel in pairs, and when they're flying solo after being torn from their mate, they'll steal electrons from other molecules in order to pair up again. Damage can be done to cell membranes, proteins, and the genetic material that guides the cell's growth and apoptosis (its appointed time to go to that big petri dish in the sky). This sets up a chain reaction that leads to cellular wear and tear and plays a role in cancer initiation and progression.

Many carcinogenic substances and behaviors trigger cancer formation by enhancing free radical production. Radiation (sunshine, X-rays, nuclear fallout), cigarette smoke, and toxins like pesticides and industrial chemicals have this effect. So do chemicals formed when meats are cooked at high temperatures or overcooked. It's interesting to note that *heterocyclic amines,* one type of chemical produced in meats cooked at high heat, are big free radical producers in the body—and they actually concentrate preferentially in the prostate gland. If you have a charred-meat habit, know that in order to enroll fully in an active holistic surveillance program, you'll have to find another way to satisfy that need. (Eating plenty of broccoli, cauliflower, and cabbage helps neutralize the effects of heterocyclic amines in the body, so if you must have that char-grilled steak, have a big heap of steamed broccoli on the side.)

The production of these free radicals is a process known as oxidation, and like inflammation, it's a natural part of the body's growth and maintenance systems. In fact, the production of free radicals is an essential part of the inflammatory process: Immune cells sent to attack pathogens do so by producing free radicals, which destroy unwanted invaders. When inflammation is chronic, a steady stream of free radicals is produced at the site of inflammation.

Nature's answer to oxidation is antioxidants—substances found in foods and made in the body that have electrons to spare. They readily donate these electrons to free radicals, neutralizing them. An antioxidant-dense diet made up primarily of whole plant foods (vegetables, fruit, whole grains, nuts, and seeds) provides a good antioxidant foundation. Certain foods like pomegranates, tomatoes, dark leafy greens, deeply colored fruits, and cruciferous vegetables (broccoli, cauliflower, and the like) are especially dense with protective antioxidants. Medicinal herbs can pack a truly superlative antioxidant punch. Supplementing with specific herbs will dramatically enhance your intake of powerful antioxidants.

At this writing, there is some controversy about whether taking high, concentrated doses of isolated antioxidant nutrients like vitamin E and vitamin C in pill form might be a bad idea for men with prostate cancer. Some studies actually suggest that high-dose antioxidants could *enhance* the formation and growth of cancer or that they could interfere with allopathic treatments. Antioxidants found in foods and herbs—in their natural forms, complexed with complementary substances that help the body utilize them efficiently—seem a safer bet at this juncture.

Foods vs. Food Supplements

When studies of populations demonstrate that people who eat lots of a certain food have lowered risk of a disease, our next goal is often to figure out what particular chemical in that food has a chemopreventive effect. This approach came from modern drug development methods. If we can determine that a single chemical compound has a "magic bullet" effect against cancer, drugmakers can manufacture something similar to it and patent it as a drug, or supplement makers can try to isolate and sell the chemical in question as a nutritional supplement.

The actual actions and effects of nutrients in foods tend to frustrate these efforts. Repeatedly, we find that when we isolate one of these ingredients and administer it in high doses, it doesn't do what we think it will, or—as many drugs do—it ends up having the opposite effect from what we intended. For example, beta-carotene, the nutrient that turns carrots orange, is a powerful antioxidant that was tested as a chemopreventive in smokers. All the evidence suggested that it would help prevent cancer in these smokers, but it had the opposite effect when taken as an isolated nutrient. It increased their risk of developing lung cancer.

The take-home lesson for the nutritional research community: The magic bullet approach is not likely to work with compounds found in the foods we eat. Most nutrients seem to need the complementary ingredients with which they exist in the whole plant or food. Although I will recommend some high-dose nutritional supplements for our chemoprevention program where research merits their use—including vitamin D and omega-3 fatty acids—they are exactly that: *supplements* to a whole-food diet.

Eating to Beat Prostate Cancer: Guys' Guidelines

If you've ever watched the cooking shows offered by the Food Network, you might have seen a few programs featuring male cooks. Now, this is a generalization, but it seems that the men offering culinary coaching on this network may not have the best interest of your prostate gland (or any other system in your body aside from your taste buds) at heart.

In his show *Diners, Drive-Ins and Dives*, portly, bleached-blond restaurateur Guy Fieri ecstatically chows down on sandwiches filled with greasy meat; macaroni and cheese with three different cheeses; eggs scrambled with more greasy meat (there's even something called a "chorizo garbage plate"); plates of just plain greasy meat; and white-flour-intensive baked goods. This isn't just Guy food, it's stereotypical American *guy* food, and if you are invested in restoring or maintaining a body that does not invite the growth or spread of cancer, it's not the kind of food you should be eating.

Overall, the best diet for prostate cancer chemoprevention most closely resembles the traditional diets of the southern Mediterranean and Japan. These diets are high in vegetables and healthful herbs. Fish and soy foods take the place of red meats, and dairy products are kept to a minimum. When oils and fats are called for, they're included in the form of oils that help reduce the omega-6 to omega-3 balance. Whole grains are favored over refined grains and foods made with flour and sugar. Both diets contain abundant fiber.

These two diets do differ in many important ways: The Mediterranean diet is rich in tomatoes, which are the best source of cancer-fighting lycopene. Its main source of fat is olive oil, which (in its extra-virgin form) is high in important antioxidants. Olive oil is high in omega-9 fatty acids, which do not promote inflammation, and contains a compound called oleocanthal that has anti-inflammatory properties. The Japanese diet includes a variety of medicinal mushrooms that have great value when it comes to cancer prevention (more on this in Chapter 9). Japanese diets also incorporate sea vegetables—a more elegant name than "seaweed." Soy foods and ginger are important parts of Japanese cuisine; Mediterranean cuisine is often flavored with rosemary and oregano. All of these foods have cancer-fighting properties.

Since we're not adhering to either the Japanese or the Mediterranean diet, we don't have to exclude any of these terrific foods from our chemoprevention suggestions. The guidelines here will help you combine the most prostate-protective characteristics of these two cuisines in a way that won't feel too exotic even for the man who has, until now, subsisted largely on fast food and frozen meals from the supermarket.

One in four Americans visits a fast-food restaurant every day. According to a survey by the Pew Charitable Trusts, most Americans choose to eat prepared or fast foods not because they taste better, but because they are more convenient.

Yes, ultimately, fast foods and prepared foods are more convenient, and they usually taste great. You'll have to face that it's never easier to make something from scratch than it is to unwrap a package and pop it in the microwave. You may need to take some time and put in some effort to learn how to prepare fresh, wholesome, delicious food at home, but it's worth it when your health and longevity hang in the balance. Changing your diet is the most important step you can take in your chemoprevention program.

Let's get the bad news out of the way first.

Chemopreventive Diet "Don'ts"

Red meat. Most studies on diet and prostate cancer have demonstrated that the more red meat a man eats, the higher his risk of developing the disease. Particularly harmful are meats that have been charred or otherwise cooked at high temperatures. If you love red meat, choose grass-fed, organic versions. Marinate in a mixture of olive oil, vinegar, and protective spices like garlic, rosemary, or turmeric, which reduces the production of carcinogenic substances during cooking.

When you do eat meat—any meat, including poultry and fish—keep servings to the size of a deck of cards or smaller.

Cured meats. Avoid cured meats like salami, bacon, lunch meat, and hot dogs, which contain cancer-encouraging nitrites.

Dairy products. Studies have found that men who consume more dairy products have a slightly higher risk of prostate cancer.

One review of 12 studies found that men who ate the most dairy had an 11 percent higher likelihood of developing prostate cancer when compared with those who ate the least dairy. This may be due to a link between prostate cancer and calcium intake, since dairy products are Americans' main source of calcium. In that same review, men with the highest intake of calcium (including calcium from nutritional supplements) had a 39 percent increased risk. Other research has found that while high intake of calcium does not seem to increase the risk of prostate cancer overall, it does seem to increase the risk of advanced or fatal prostate cancer. And some research shows that there is no relationship at all between dairy and calcium consumption and prostate cancer of any kind. The jury's still out on this one. For now, I recommend keeping dairy products to a minimum. If you love dairy, include it for flavor, but cut your usual amount by half or more.

One dairy food I often recommend is yogurt, because of the beneficial bacteria it contains. Choose organic yogurt and limit intake to a cup per day.

Saturated and trans fats. In the standard American diet, main sources of saturated fat are meats, egg yolks, and dairy products. Coconut oil, palm kernel oil, and cottonseed oil are also high in saturated fats. If a fat is solid at room temperature, consider it saturated. Trans fats are found in highly processed vegetable oils that have been bombarded with hydrogen atoms to make them fluffy solids at room temperature, which increases their shelf life and improves their texture for use as an ingredient in baked goods. Both these types of fat are linked with increased risk of heart disease and several cancers.

What's the link? With trans fats, a direct effect on prostate cancer risk has been found. All authorities agree that these fake fats should be avoided completely. The picture with saturated fats is slightly less clear. Our best guess is that saturated fats are not intrinsically carcinogenic. The issue at hand is likely to involve chemical toxins found in most sources of saturated fat, put there by modern factory farming methods. Toxins that can raise cancer risk concentrate in the fat of animals who eat a diet laced with pesticides and herbicides. Even higher concentrations of these toxins accumulate in dairy products and eggs.

Obesity, Inflammation, and Oxidation

Men who are obese have a heightened risk of developing prostate cancer, particularly the more aggressive forms of the disease. In part, this increased risk is related to changes in hormone balance characteristic of men who are carrying around 30 or more excess pounds. Another hazard of obesity—one that increases risks of all cancers, as well as heart disease—is that it exacerbates both inflammation and oxidation in the body. Obese men are also more likely to have high insulin levels and high blood sugar levels, which are precursors to type 2 diabetes. Both these circumstances accelerate inflammation and oxidation even further.

If you are a man who knows he could stand to lose a few pounds, putting my dietary guidelines into action will likely bring about weight loss. Exercise daily. Keep track of calories in and calories out and make a point of expending more than you take in on most days (see the box on page 156 for instructions on calculating caloric need). Solicit help from your doctor or from a weight loss program to try to shed some of the extra pounds you're carrying around.

Completely avoid trans fats. If a food label states that it contains "partially hydrogenated" or "hydrogenated" oils, assume that it contains trans fats, even if the label says it contains zero grams of the stuff. (Labeling requirements dictate that if less than half a gram is present per serving, the label can say that it doesn't contain any.) Minimize saturated fat intake, and if you do choose to eat foods that contain saturated fats, shop for organic, free-range versions. It will cost more, but you can just eat smaller portions.

Calculating Basal Metabolic Rate and Caloric Need

Basal metabolic rate (BMR) is the number of calories you require to maintain your weight if you do absolutely nothing all day but lie around.

If you measure your weight in pounds and height in inches, use this formula:

$$BMR = 66 + (6.23 \times \text{weight in pounds}) + (12.7 \times \text{height in inches}) - (6.8 \times \text{age in years})$$

If you measure your weight in kilograms and your height in centimeters, use this formula:

$$BMR = 66 + (13.7 \times \text{weight in kilograms}) + (5 \times \text{height in centimeters}) - (6.8 \times \text{age in years})$$

Then, take that BMR and plug it into the *Harris-Benedict equation,* which allows you to calculate caloric requirements based on your physical activity level.

• If you're sedentary, multiply BMR by 1.2.

• If you do light activity or sports 1 to 2 days a week, multiply BMR by 1.375.

Foods high in white flour and sugars. Sugars fan the flames of chronic inflammation. The body responds to refined flour in much the same way it responds to sugar, so it's sensible to minimize intake of both. The low-fat diets once recommended for weight loss and health promotion tended to be high in these exact foods, and the result was a population that chronically craved refined carbohydrates (because without some fat and protein, blood sugars rise and crash, leading to more carb cravings) and

---

- If you do moderate exercise or sports 3 to 5 days a week, multiply BMR by 1.55.

- If you do moderate or hard exercise 6 to 7 days a week, multiply BMR by 1.725.

- If you are extra-active, with hard activity once or twice a day or a physical job, multiply BMR by 1.9.

Once you've figured out your daily caloric needs, check online for a calorie calculator that works for you. Some cell phone applications and computer programs feature calorie counters and journals for food record keeping. Or if you're more old school, buy a calorie-counting book. From there, it's simple: Try to eat about the same number of calories you expend if you're trying to maintain weight; try to eat fewer if you want to lose weight. If you eat according to the guidelines laid out here, you're not likely to have any trouble staying within your caloric limits—even if you cheat once in a while, as everyone does. (Someone wise once said, "Everything in moderation . . . including moderation.") If you blow it one day, make up for it in the days following. No need to be hard on yourself.

Note that your caloric needs will decrease as you get older. Recalculate every couple of years.

ended up fatter than they would have if they had created a more balanced diet. Obesity and a diet heavy in refined carbs is a direct cause of insulin resistance, a precursor to type 2 diabetes. None of this bodes well for a man's prostate; it exacerbates both inflammation and oxidative stress.

When you eat grains, choose them in a form as close as possible to the ones in which they occur in nature: brown rice instead of white and whole-grain or sprouted-grain crackers and breads, for example. Whole grains in the diet have an inverse relationship with prostate cancer risk. They're rich in fiber that helps remove carcinogens from the body.

Smoked, pickled, or overly salted foods. While these foods haven't been linked directly to prostate cancer, they have been linked to stomach and colorectal cancers. They are best eaten in extreme moderation.

That's the full picture of foods to avoid for the sake of chemo-prevention. And now for the good news. . . .

Chemopreventive Diet "Dos"

Eat mindfully. Believe it or not, the first step to making big shifts in your diet is becoming more *conscious* about what you eat. If you prefer a less esoteric way of describing it, start paying attention to what you're putting in your mouth.

Notice your eating habits—not what you eat, but *how* you eat. Do you tend to wait until you're famished, then toss as much food as possible down your throat in one sitting? Does this habit lead you to choose foods you know are not healthy for you or to eat until you're overfull? Do you often eat in your car or at your desk? Do you pay attention to the taste of your food and chew it thoroughly?

Being mindful while you eat will help you slow down in the course of your busy day, which will reduce stress. It will help you be more aware of how much you're eating and give you an enhanced awareness of the point at which you're full. You're all grown up now; you don't have to clean your plate.

Eating consciously means savoring your food, which will reduce cravings for intensely flavored sweet, salty, and fatty junk and enhance your taste buds' appreciation of healthy whole foods. Chewing food thoroughly (until it's liquid in your mouth) will mean fewer gastrointestinal complaints.

Reduce calories consumed. Many, many studies have found that the simple act of eating too many calories raises cancer risk, while underconsuming calories reduces it. A few researchers have demonstrated amazing age-delaying and anti-cancer effects in animals fed 30 percent less than they would eat if they were given free access to food.

Human beings with free will are highly unlikely to opt for a diet like this one, since it means being hungry all the time. But an awareness of roughly the number of calories you take in versus the number you expend will help reduce excess fat, which reduces inflammation and improves hormone balance.

Eat fish. Flesh foods, eggs, and milk used to have a better omega-6/omega-3 balance when the land animals we ate— chickens, cows—grazed on omega-3-rich grass in the fields instead of eating omega-6-rich corn, as they do today. As it is now, your best food bet for a high omega-3 content is fish.

Fish is the best dietary source of the omega-3 fats DHA (docosahexaenoic acid) and EPA (eicosapentaenoic acid). Eating fish (one serving is about the size of a deck of playing cards) one to two times a week will help balance out that all-important omega-6/omega-3 ratio. Whenever possible, choose wild-caught, high-omega-3 fish like salmon and sardines. The colder the water the fish lives in, the more omega-3 oils its flesh contains; since omega-3 oils don't freeze, high content prevents these fish from freezing solid. Choose cold-water fish when you can.

Fish farming and overfishing practices have caused concern about the sustainability of seafood populations; so have indications that fish can become contaminated with neurotoxic mercury and carcinogenic industrial chemicals. The higher a fish is on the food chain, the more likely it is to have concentrated chemicals and mercury in its meat, so eat as low on the marine food chain as possible. Wild-caught fish is generally less likely to contain toxins, but in some cases fish farming creates a sustainable source of seafood that is acceptable as an omega-3 source.

According to *U.S. News & World Report*, the 10 best fish choices are wild Alaskan salmon, Arctic char (farmed is okay), Atlantic mackerel, sardines (Andrew Weil, MD, suggests mashing oil-packed sardines with onion and mustard to make a spread), sablefish/black cod, anchovies, oysters, rainbow trout (children should not eat more than two or three meals of this fish per month owing to concerns about polychorinated biphenyls, aka PCBs), tuna (limit to three meals a month), and mussels. A good current source for information on safe, sustainable fish is the Monterey Bay Aquarium's Web site: http://www.montereybayaquarium.org/cr/seafood-watch.aspx.

Add as many vegetables as possible to meals and snacks. Here is your mission, should you accept it: Cram as many vegetables as possible into every meal and snack you consume. Try chopping onions, tomatoes, peppers, or chard and sautéing them in olive oil, then adding eggs and scrambling. Chop spinach, broccoli, or other vegetables and add to soups (baby spinach can be thrown into hot broth raw; it will blanch just enough to be cooked through). Eat one large green salad a day with a dressing of olive oil and vinegar.

Try doubling up on vegetables, and halve the size of refined carbohydrate and protein servings. In restaurants, order a side of steamed vegetables or coleslaw instead of fries or rice. Hit every color and type of vegetable you can—the more colorful the better, as deeper color usually means greater antioxidant nutrition.

Of course, this is going to feel punishing if you eat iceberg lettuce and steamed broccoli every day. Experiment with vegetables you might not have tried before. Go to the farmer's market or to a store that carries lots of fresh, seasonal, organic vegetables. Try sea vegetables, which are a mainstay of Japanese cuisine; they're highly nutrient-dense and flavorful. Whip up veggie-rich meals with people you love. Look at it as a culinary adventure.

Consume vegetables raw, lightly steamed, baked, roasted, sautéed, in soups, or stir-fried. If you want to amp up their taste, try adding small amounts of flavorful cheese, sauces, herbs, and spices. The bioavailability of lycopene in tomatoes is maximized by cooking with olive oil. Avoid fried vegetables (French fries included) or vegetables dipped in batter and deep-fried.

Concentrate on crucifers. In particular, include broccoli, cauliflower, cabbage, Brussels sprouts, and kale, all of which belong to the family of cruciferous vegetables. They contain *isothiocyanates* and *sulforaphane*, chemicals that have been found to impact cancer initiation, angiogenesis (the process by which tumors sprout their own circulatory systems, facilitating their growth and spread), and the body's ability to neutralize carcinogenic substances. Phytochemicals from cruciferous vegetables also reduce body levels of harmful estrogens by encouraging their conversion to less harmful forms.

Go for greens. Also emphasize deeply colored leafy greens like spinach, salad greens, and Swiss chard, which are especially rich in antioxidant vitamins, minerals, and phytochemicals; sprouts of every sort, broccoli sprouts in particular; and tomatoes, which are high in lycopene, an antioxidant believed to help reduce prostate cancer risk.

Sacrifice fresh breath for a healthy prostate. Allium-family vegetables like onions, leeks, scallions, shallots, chives, and garlic have been used throughout most of human history for medicinal purposes. Modern science shows that they are antimicrobial and antiarthritic as well as helpful for maintaining healthy blood sugar balance, joint health, and blood cholesterol levels. They contain multiple antioxidant and anti-cancer substances, including the bioflavonoid *quercetin,* the anti-cancer mineral *selenium,* and *organosulfur compounds.* Organosulfur compounds support detoxification of carcinogens, inhibit tumor cell proliferation, scavenge free radicals, inhibit DNA changes that lead to cancer, slow cancer cell growth, and induce apoptosis.

Dive into deeply colored fruits like pomegranates, red grapes, and blueberries . . . and enjoy red wine. Deeply colored red and purple fruits are rich in *ellagitannins* and other compounds with antioxidant and anti-inflammatory actions in the body. Cranberries were found in one study to enhance prostate

How to Eat a Fresh Pomegranate

Getting at the edible parts of a fresh pomegranate can be a messy challenge; if you try to slice it open with a knife, bloodred juice squirts out as you cut into the arils. Here's how to do it neatly.

Turn the fruit with the stem end up. Use a slim, sharp knife to cut around the place where the stem was attached to the fruit. Lift out the stem attachment, then push your thumbs into the opening you've just created and crack open the fruit. Break it into sections and gently pull the arils out of the skin.

cancer cell apoptosis. The two most exciting lines of study regarding fruits and prostate cancer chemoprevention involve red grapes and pomegranate.

Research at the MD Anderson Cancer Center in Texas has found that tumors may become *chemosensitized*—made more vulnerable to standard chemotherapy medicines—when exposed to the antioxidant, anti-inflammatory chemical *resveratrol*. Red grape skins and seeds are a good source of resveratrol, as is red wine. More will be said about resveratrol in Chapter 8, when we look at herbal chemopreventives. For now, add dark-colored grapes to your diet—they make a good substitute for more processed sweets. Or enjoy a glass of red wine a few days a week.

Pomegranates are an especially promising nutritional chemopreventive for men with prostate cancer. The ruby red seeds, or *arils,* of this fruit contain abundant *epigallocatechin gallate,* a compound also found in green tea, *delphinidin chloride, kaempferol,* and *punicic acid,* all of which have been found to inhibit cell growth spurred by dihydrotestosterone. Pomegranate is also rich in antioxidant *tannins* and *flavonoids*. In fact, measurement of the antioxidant activity of pomegranate juice found that it has about 18 to 20 times the antioxidant power of red wine and green tea. Other effects of pomegranate/pomegranate juice found in test-tube studies: induction of apoptosis, slowing of cancer cell growth, and inhibition of prostate cancer cell invasion. One study found that men who drank pomegranate juice after being diagnosed with prostate cancer prolonged PSA doubling time significantly.

Add pomegranate to your diet in juice form, or eat the arils fresh. The arils are tart-sweet and are good on their own or tossed into a green salad.

Incorporate soy foods in moderation. Soy foods are the richest dietary source of *isoflavones*, plant chemicals that have been found to directly inhibit the growth of cancer cells in laboratory studies. Isoflavones act as weak estrogens and have apoptotic and antiangiogenic effects. Surveys of tens of thousands of Japanese men suggest that soy foods reduce the risk of developing localized prostate cancer, but they may not help reduce the risk of advanced prostate cancer. In other words, we don't yet know enough about the effects of soy isoflavones on all varieties of prostate cancer to recommend piling on the soy in excess with soy protein powders, tofu, and soy milk. We do know enough to suggest that including a moderate serving or two of soy a day can help protect against dying from the disease.

Try nuts and seeds, including walnuts and flaxseed (but not flaxseed oil). Research has demonstrated that men whose diets include more nuts and seeds have a lowered risk of developing prostate cancer. Nuts and seeds are great sources of healthy fats, fiber, and the antioxidant vitamin E. In one study, rats genetically engineered to develop prostate cancer were fed standard high-fat diets where fat came from soy oil or diets supplemented with walnuts to equal the same amount of calories from fat. The walnut-eating rats had slower tumor growth than rats who ate the standard diet.

Flaxseed is a superior source of a particular kind of fiber known as *lignan;* it contains some 800 times more lignan than other foods! Lignan has antiangiogenic and antioxidant effects. It acts as a weak estrogen that helps to block prostate cancer's growth in response to stronger estrogens and testosterone, and it has even been found to block the enzyme that transforms testosterone into its more active form, dihydrotestosterone. In one study, men supplemented with ground flaxseed for 30 days before prostate cancer surgery had less prostate cancer cell growth than men who did not take flaxseed. Flaxseeds can be consumed in ground form mixed with yogurt, hot cereals, or smoothies.

Flaxseeds and walnuts are high in omega-3 fats, but they don't replace EPA and DHA from fish oils. The omega-3s found in flax and walnuts are short-chain fatty acids called alpha-linolenic acid (ALA), and in order to match the anti-inflammatory power of EPA and DHA, they have to be converted into these longer-chain fatty acids. Conversion can be inefficient, so it's unwise to rely on ALA to fulfill your need for anti-inflammatory omega-3s.

Drink more tea (including green tea), pomegranate juice, and purified water. Stay away from sodas—even diet sodas, which have not been found to help with weight loss—and try more healthful beverages. Green tea is available in just about every flavor; sweeten with a small amount of honey or agave or the herb stevia. Pomegranate juice is high in sugar, so feel free to chase it (or dilute it) with water.

Diet Is More Important Than Supplements for Chemoprevention!

The chemopreventive diet doesn't include a bunch of recipes, "points," or even precise serving sizes for most of what it contains. This is because it's not really about the quantity of food you eat; it's about the quality. It's about changing your food staples and doing so permanently. And in avoiding the "don'ts" and adhering to the "dos," you'll learn to cook, eat, and enjoy food in a new way. Guy Fieri may not want to have what you're having, but in the end, your prostate (and your loved ones, who want you to live a long, healthy life) will be the better for these shifts.

In the next chapter, I'll cover a complete nutritional supplement program for chemoprevention. Before you move on, consider how in our culture we like to think that we can cancel out the negative impact of a lousy diet by popping a few pills. This is wishful thinking. Whether it contains powerful pharmaceuticals or rain forest herbs, any pill will do its job better when taken in the context of a truly healthy, balanced diet rich in vegetables, fruit, healthy oils, and whole grains. The truth is that if you don't adhere to the diet guidelines in this chapter, the supplements in the following chapter will probably not make nearly as much difference.

CHAPTER 9

MUCH MORE THAN ROOTS, LEAVES, AND BERRIES: THE CENTER FOR HOLISTIC UROLOGY'S HERBAL AND NUTRITIONAL SUPPLEMENT RECOMMENDATIONS

If you walk into a health food store to shop for supplements without any guidance beforehand, or if you go online and do a Google search for "prostate+supplements," you're going to be overwhelmed, fast. Now that you understand the main prostate cancer mechanisms we can control with nutritional medicine, let's talk practicalities.

The supplements we recommend in the Center for Holistic Urology's chemoprevention program will almost all help to reduce inflammation or oxidation. The program's recommended diet shifts and herbal and nutritional medicines have other benefits as well, including:

- forestalling *angiogenesis,* the process by which tumors sprout their very own circulatory systems to aid in their growth and spread

- accelerating *apoptosis,* or programmed cell death, preferentially suppressing cancer cell growth

- directly affecting DNA in ways that inhibit cancer formation

- promoting better liver function, which helps the body to neutralize carcinogens

- affecting hormone levels in the body in ways that reduce testosterone and estrogen effects on prostate cancer cells

Start with a *multivitamin/mineral* supplement, preferably one that contains nutrients in "whole food" form rather than as isolated, lab-created vitamins and minerals. Avoid megadoses hundreds or thousands of times beyond the recommended daily intake. When nutrients are in whole-food form, they are absorbed and utilized more efficiently than they are as isolated nutrients made in a laboratory; megadoses aren't needed to get adequate nutrients into the cells where they can be used. Think of the multivitamin as a kind of insurance against any dietary deficiencies that might negatively impact your health.

Add to your "multi":

Vitamin D. You might know vitamin D as the "sunshine vitamin" that the body can make during exposure to sunlight. Vitamin D is also found in foods, most abundantly in fish and in dairy products to which the vitamin has been added. This vitamin helps to regulate cell growth, cell death, and cell differentiation, all of which help dictate whether cancer develops and spreads. Studies show that men who live in parts of the world that get less sunshine may be at greater risk of developing prostate cancer. Darker-skinned men are less able to produce vitamin D in their skin; if vitamin D plays a role in protecting against prostate cancer, this helps to make sense of the much higher risk seen in African Americans. Genetic differences in the body's efficiency at processing and using vitamin D seem correlated to genes that confer increased risk of prostate cancer.

Research in both laboratory and population settings shows that adequate vitamin D both reduces the risk of prostate cancer (and other cancers) and may help to slow its growth in men who have already developed the disease. One large study found that men who have higher levels of sun exposure during recreational activities halve their risk of dying of prostate cancer. Another study—the second phase of the Physicians' Health Study, which enrolled almost 15,000 men and investigated how their lifestyles, diets, and habits impacted their risk of various health problems—found that two-thirds of the subjects had low vitamin D levels in the spring and winter, when the sun's rays are least strong in North America. Of men who ended up developing prostate cancer, those with the lowest blood vitamin D levels were the most likely to have an aggressive form of the disease—especially if they were over 65. This makes sense when we consider that the ability to produce vitamin D and to utilize the nutrient when consumed in foods decreases with age. Another study found that vitamin D supplements reduced or stabilized PSA in about 20 percent of a group of 26 men with asymptomatic prostate cancer that had spread beyond the gland.

When I lecture about alternative medicine to urologists, I usually ask how many of them obtain vitamin D levels as part of their routine patient tests. When only a few hands go up, as is almost always the case, I let them know that I believe there is enough information in the literature and enough research to support measuring vitamin D levels in men who are at risk for this disease. At Columbia University Medical Center, we tested the vitamin D levels of over 3,000 urology patients and found that nearly 70 percent of the men were deficient in vitamin D. The paper we wrote about this finding, which will be published in the *Journal of Urology*, may influence urological practices around the world. If your urologist or another physician is willing to test your vitamin D, have him or her do so; if the level is below normal, start to take vitamin D_3 supplements daily. I recommend starting out with 5,000 IU a day and then repeating the vitamin D test after 3 months' use of the supplement. The goal is to get to blood levels above 50 ng/ml (125 nmol/L) and keep them there year-round.

Fifteen minutes of direct sunshine (without sunscreen) on your hands and face makes about twice this much in Caucasian skin. Darker-skinned people need about 45 minutes of direct sun to produce a day's worth of vitamin D, which could help explain why risk is so much higher in African Americans. Supplementing at the dose I'm recommending is completely safe; you'd have to take 40,000 IU a day for quite a while to reach the point of toxicity.

Fish oils. To control chronic inflammation, I suggest that men create a desirable balance between omega-6 and omega-3 fats. The ideal ratio between omega-6 and omega-3 is 2 to 1; most Americans eat diets with ratios that far exceed this, ranging from 10 to 1 to as high as 30 to 1. Blood samples taken from American men have shown that the typical Western diet creates a balance of about 80 percent omega-6 and 20 percent omega-3 in the body. In the prostate-protective Mediterranean diet, this is almost reversed. This fatty acid balance in our bodies is very important; even slight rises in the omega-6/omega-3 ratio are associated with a higher risk of diseases like arthritis and cancer.

Omega-6/omega-3 ratio can now be determined with a simple finger-stick blood test. The result is analyzed by several labs. It's good to know this ratio for yourself, because the higher it is, the greater your risk of chronic inflammation. As you modify your diet, you can retest and see the ratio changing—and know that in the process, you're reducing your risk by modifying some of the genes that are turned on during cancer development. Dietary shifts will help to reduce this ratio, but I also advise men on a chemopreventive protocol to add supplemental omega-3 fats by taking fish oil.

According to a review of studies authored by a group at Duke University, the highest ratio of omega-6 to omega-3 intake is strongly associated with increased risk of high-grade prostate cancer (but not low-grade prostate cancer). Test-tube studies have shown that one omega-3 fatty acid in particular, DHA, selectively induces prostate cancer cells to become more sensitive to attack by the body's own immune defenses.

Choose a fish oil derived from wild-caught fish. Salmon, sardines, and anchovies are good choices that are unlikely to be contaminated with unwanted chemicals or heavy metals. I recommend getting 1-4 grams per day of the omega-3 DHA and EPA combined. This equips the body with raw materials needed to reduce the production of pro-inflammatory eicosanoids and to enhance the production of anti-inflammatory eicosanoids.

If you prefer a vegetarian source of EPA and DHA, supplements made from algae—the food source of these fats for fish—are available.

Zyflamend. When I suggest my patients use herbs, I'm not talking about any old herb from the health food store shelf. Studies performed to test these natural substances have used versions of these plants that are (almost always) organic and *standardized* (processed in a way that ensures an adequate content of active constituents).

At the Center for Holistic Urology, we have extensively researched Zyflamend, a supplement made from the extracts of 10 herbs with known anti-inflammatory effects. We've looked particularly at its potential both as a chemopreventive agent that can be used in men who have chosen active holistic surveillance and as part of an overall plan to prevent recurrence in men who have undergone treatment. This product is made by a company called New Chapter in Brattleboro, Vermont.

At the Center for Holistic Urology, we gave Zyflamend to 23 men with PIN (prostatic intraepithelial neoplasia, a precancerous condition that can turn into prostate cancer) for 18 months. The men had blood drawn every 3 months so that PSA and other blood chemistries could be measured. Every 6 months, the men repeated the biopsy. No man had any serious side effects or toxicity; some had mild gastrointestinal complaints while taking the supplement. Just under half of the subjects had a 25 to 50 percent decrease in PSA after 18 months on Zyflamend. Nine of 15 who had the final biopsy (attrition is a normal part of doing these studies) had all benign tissue with no sign of PIN. Four of 15 still had PIN in one core. Biopsies of the remaining 2 of these 15 men showed that small, insignificant cancers had developed.

At the University of Texas, researchers studied the molecular effects of Zyflamend in samples of prostate cancer. They found that this combination of herbs inhibits invasion of cancer cells, reduces the ability of cancer to spread to bone cells, and boosts apoptosis through anti-inflammatory effects on cells' genetic blueprints.

I don't mean to endorse any particular brand of herbal supplement. It isn't imperative that you choose Zyflamend to get the benefits of the herbs it contains—you can take them all separately if you prefer or find another product that contains some of the same ingredients, such as ProstaCaid, a similar product we've also researched at the Center for Holistic Urology (see "Prostacaid" on page 78). But the research we've done in our labs and our investigations into what this company is doing have convinced me that Zyflamend is a high-quality product that effectively reins in chronic inflammation. New Chapter's method of concentrating whole herbs into supercritical extracts—essentially highly concentrated, complete versions of the natural herb—seems to create a superior product. I recommend New Chapter's products, particularly Zyflamend, to all of my patients who are interested in chemoprevention.

Zyflamend contains:

- 150 mg **rosemary leaf** extract, standardized to 34.5 mg total phenolic antioxidants.

Rosemary, an important flavoring herb in the Mediterranean diet, contains two compounds with special promise for chemoprevention: *carnosic acid* and *rosmarinic acid*. These compounds are antibacterial and have very strong antioxidant activity. Consuming this herb not only raises antioxidant intake, it also potentiates the body's production of its own antioxidant substances.

- 110 mg **turmeric** extract, standardized to 4.5 mg turmerones and 7 mg curcuminoids.

This Asian spice belongs to the same family as the ginger-root. Owing to its anti-infective, anti-inflammatory, and digestion-soothing properties, turmeric has been used in Ayurvedic (Asian Indian) and Chinese medicine for over 4,000 years to treat a broad variety of health problems, including arthritis, wounds, liver disease, digestive disorders, diabetes, and cancer.

Studies of turmeric's effects on isolated cancer cells and on animals demonstrate that its active ingredient, *curcumin*, inhibits tumor initiation and proliferation in almost every type of cancer. Modern test-tube studies show that curcumin reduces levels of the COX-2 and LOX enzymes that produce pro-inflammatory eicosanoids. Many of the steps that create and foster the growth of cancer involve inflammation, and turmeric suppresses several of them, reducing cancer cell proliferation and increasing cancer cell death. Turmeric also acts as a powerful antioxidant. Some research even finds that curcumin helps reduce the inflammatory state that tends to accompany obesity.

Turmeric helps reduce excessive blood clotting and aids in balancing cholesterol counts, which promotes better heart health; it reduces blood sugar levels in diabetics; and some studies even find that it protects the brain against age-related degeneration.

This herb shows so much promise as a chemopreventive

agent that I recommend men take a bit extra in addition to what is found in Zyflamend. New Chapter makes a supplement called Turmericforce, which contains 400 mg turmeric (minimum 22 mg curcuminoids).

● 100 mg **ginger** extract, standardized to 16.2 mg pungent compounds and 4.3 mg zingiberene.

Gingerroot, with its anti-inflammatory, anti-nausea, and anti-infective properties, has been used as a remedy in traditional medicine for thousands of years. It helps soothe coughs and is one of the best palliatives for motion sickness. Ginger's active compounds—*gingerols* and *shogaols*—work as natural COX-2 inhibitors and antioxidants.

● 100 mg **holy basil** extract.

Also known as tulsi, tulasi, and *Ocimum tenuiflorum,* holy basil is an ancient Ayurvedic medicinal plant that, like turmeric, has been avidly researched for its chemopreventive potential. Its active components, including *eugenol, carvacrol, oleanolic acid,* and *ursolic acid,* inhibit COX-2, act as strong antioxidants, and help reduce blood sugar levels. Studies demonstrate that holy basil down-regulates growth-promoting processes that otherwise facilitate cancer cell growth. It is antimetastatic, inhibiting cancer cell invasion and adhesion, and it increases cancer cells' susceptibility to death by chemotherapy.

I advise patients to take New Chapter's Holy Basil supplement in addition to Zyflamend. Each serving of two capsules contains 800 mg of the herb, standardized to 2 percent ursolic acid.

● 100 mg **green tea** leaf extract, standardized to 45 mg polyphenols.

Tea is a rich source of *catechins*, which belong to a class of medicinal plant compounds called polyphenols. Green tea is the best-known source of the catechin *epigallocatechin gallate*, or EGCG for short. Catechins protect against cellular damage caused by oxidative stress and modify several metabolic and cell-signaling pathways that regulate cancer cell growth, spread, and survival. Tea polyphenols have beneficial effects along the whole spectrum of cancer formation, growth, and spread, affecting apoptosis, angiogenesis, and metastasis in ways that aid in chemoprevention.

One study of smokers found that giving smokers green tea daily reduced by 50 percent the formation of *DNA adducts*— abnormal sections of DNA that predispose the cell to becoming cancerous. Green tea polyphenols also appear to directly affect the body's processing of cancer-causing substances, reducing the expression of enzymes that would otherwise interact with carcinogens in ways that make them more carcinogenic. Specific to the prostate, research has shown that green tea administration inhibited the development of cancerous cells from precancerous lesions (such as PIN).

I suggest drinking green tea regularly. Black and white teas are also beneficial, so drink them too if you like. New Chapter Organics Green & White Tea Force supplement can be taken by men who don't like tea. It contains a minimum of 40 percent polyphenols and 12 percent EGCG. Stick with caffeinated versions if you tolerate caffeine well. Caffeine naturally present in tea is believed to play a role in its chemopreventive effects.

- 80 mg **Hu zhang** (*Polygonum cuspidatum*), standardized to 6.4 mg resveratrol.

Hu zhang, also known as Japanese knotweed, is a traditional Chinese herb that happens to be naturally rich in the phytochemical *resveratrol*—the antioxidant present in red grapes and in red wine. Studies demonstrate that resveratrol-rich hu zhang reduces inflammation and oxidative stress through several different mechanisms; in fact, it seems to affect every step of cancer formation and spread—initiation, promotion, and progression—as well as suppressing angiogenesis and metastasis. Resveratrol also blocks the transformation of less harmful catechol estrogens into more carcinogenic quinone estrogens and triggers apoptosis.

- 40 mg each **Chinese goldthread** and **barberry,** each standardized to contain 2.4 mg berberine.

These two traditional Chinese herbs, both of which have been used medicinally for at least two and a half millennia, are rich sources of a plant chemical called berberine. Berberine inhibits activities in cells' metabolic "engines" (mitochondria) that can promote carcinogenic transformation. It also reduces the expression of the COX-2 enzyme, which means less inflammation. In test-tube studies of prostate cancer cells, berberine inhibited cell growth by inducing apoptosis. Several other survival schemes mounted by cancer cells are thwarted by berberine, which is a hot subject of research in chemoprevention circles.

- 40 mg **oregano** extract, standardized to 1.6 mg total phenolic antioxidants.

  This Mediterranean herb has high antioxidant activity thanks to its dense content of plant chemicals known as phenolic acids and flavonoids. Studies suggest that oregano is selectively toxic to tumor cells. It is a rich source of *quercetin,* an antioxidant, anti-inflammatory flavonoid.

- 20 mg **Baikal skullcap** (*Scutellaria baicalensis*) extract, standardized to 3.4 mg baicalein complex, including baicalein and baicalin, and 0.08 mg wogonin.

ProstaCaid: Another Promising Herbal Combination for Chemoprevention

At the Center for Holistic Urology, we studied the effects on prostate cancer cell lines of ProstaCaid (EcoNugenics, Santa Rosa, California), a blend of 33 different ingredients, including vitamins, minerals, and multiple herb extracts from the same plants used in the making of Zyflamend. The supplement inhibited the growth of both human and mouse prostate cancer cells, both androgen-dependent (those that need testosterone to grow) and androgen-independent (those that grow in the absence of testosterone). When we looked at the effects of ProstaCaid at the molecular level, we found many ways in which it impacted cancer cell growth: reduction of prostate cancer cell colony formation after long-term treatment, for example, as well as increased apoptosis. Although we haven't yet done as much research into this supplement as we have with others, ProstaCaid appears to have potential for chemoprevention—perhaps even as an adjunct therapy for men with androgen-independent prostate cancer.

Yet another Chinese herb that packs a big antioxidant, anti-inflammatory punch. Test-tube studies show that it inhibits the action of the COX-2 enzyme, which then decreases production of the inflammatory eicosanoid prostaglandin E2. Animal studies have shown dramatic effects of Baikal skullcap on cancer growth: One study showed a 50 percent reduction in prostate tumor volume in animals given skullcap for 7 weeks, while another showed a 66 percent reduction! Wogonin, an active constituent of skullcap, was found in one study to block the production of an enzyme in cancer cells that is needed for survival. As a result of this blockade, the cancer cells committed suicide (apoptosis).

Because this herb seems so promising as a chemopreventive, I recommend that men use New Chapter's Chinese Skullcap on its own in addition to what's found in Zyflamend. The supplement contains 200 mg of extract per dose, standardized to 34 mg baicalein complex and 0.8 mg wogonin.

Medicinal Mushrooms

Even the plain white button mushrooms at your local grocery store are full of nutrients important for human health. They are rich in the B vitamins niacin, riboflavin, and pantothenic acid and in the minerals potassium and selenium. Selenium is a nutrient that has been studied for its anti-cancer and antioxidant properties. Research has shown that men who consume the most dietary selenium have about half the risk of developing advanced prostate cancer compared with men who consume the least.

Medicinal mushrooms have been a subject of intensive research in cancer chemoprevention. Two medicinal mushrooms, *Coprinus comatus* and *Ganoderma lucidum*, have been found to act as natural antiandrogenic modulators. The medicinal mushroom *reishi*, which has been used as a chemotherapy agent since ancient China, inhibits inflammation and appears to reduce the invasiveness and metastatic potential of breast and prostate tumors. Reishi's bioactive ingredients seem to be strong contenders as chemopreventives. There is no evidence that use of medicinal mushrooms has a downside in terms of chemoprevention.

In our holistic urology protocol, we use a supplement called AHCC (active hexose correlated compound), which is a combination of several species of medicinal mushrooms. A study of healthy adults 50 years of age and up found that AHCC supplementation improved T-cell immune response, which aids in resistance against the development and spread of cancer. Other research points to the value of AHCC in enhancing cell differentiation (remember that cancer cells are *un*differentiated—the more undifferentiated, the more dangerous the cancer). AHCC has antioxidant effects and enhances *tumor surveillance,* the body's ability to detect and attack cancerous cells.

To date, most of the many studies of this fermented blend of Japanese mushrooms show that it enhances components within the immune system that are known to fight a variety of cancers, including gastric, hepatic, breast, and prostate. Studies also show that AHCC can reduce side effects in patients undergoing chemotherapy.

This supplement is a mainstay in our program. The dose for

low-stage disease differs from that for higher stages. For low-risk prostate cancer, I suggest 3 grams a day; if your PSA is higher, I recommend 5 grams a day. The product is produced in Japan by a company called Amino Up and is imported into the United States by Quality of Life labs. You should be able to find it at your local health food store as well as online.

CHAPTER 10

WORKING OUT
AND CHILLING OUT:
TWO SIDES OF THE SAME
CHEMOPREVENTIVE COIN

According to the 2009 National Health Interview Survey, 65 percent of adults over the age of 18 do not engage in regular leisure-time physical activity. In the same survey, 55 percent of adults had never in their lives engaged in regular physical activity! If you belong to either of these demographics and want to increase your chances of living a life that won't end because of prostate cancer, it's time for you, old dog, to start doing some new tricks.

As rare as a regular exercise program is for most men, rarer still is the use of meditation, yoga, or a support group. Most men who get to the point of integrating stress reduction techniques do so because of an urgent health issue . . . like prostate cancer or a prostate cancer scare. Still, the average guy who knuckles under and commits to a stress reduction program is usually very glad he did; his quality of life and general health improve, and he wonders why he didn't check out this stress reduction stuff sooner. The fact is that a man who incorporates both stress reduction and regular exercise has a better chance of beating prostate cancer than the man who incorporates only one or the other. And if you modify your diet in the ways advised in Chapter 8, your chances are better still. These three interventions work best when mounted all at once.

Important as exercise is, stress reduction is just as essential for overall good health and cancer prevention and control. A life high in stress and low on relaxation creates physiological changes that increase the risk of developing cancer and many other ailments, including cardiovascular disease and gastrointestinal problems.

In this chapter, you'll learn in more detail why exercise and stress reduction are (as the chapter title indicates) two sides of the same chemopreventive coin. Yes, incorporating just one—exercise or stress reduction—is beneficial, but adding both to your life will give you the best of both worlds.

All of the guidelines given in this chapter should help to reduce your risk of developing prostate cancer. However, the men who stand to benefit most from exercise and stress reduction are those who are diagnosed with PIN or are advised to watch and wait—in holistic urology terms, those who are engaged in active holistic surveillance.

Studies Confirm That Lifestyle Modification Helps Stop Prostate Cancer Progression

A research team at the University of California in San Francisco has conducted a series of studies on men with low-risk prostate cancer who either had no intervention with respect to diet, exercise, or stress reduction (the control group) or had all three interventions—the so-called lifestyle modification program. This program, created by Dean Ornish, MD, was first made famous in its application for treating heart disease, where it was found to reverse the atherosclerosis (clogging of arteries) that leads to heart attack.

Six men in the control group went into conventional treatment during the course of the study because their prostate cancer had progressed. In the lifestyle modification group, PSA dropped 4 percent, while the men in the control group saw a rise of 6 percent. Over the course of 1 year, none of the men in the lifestyle modification program required conventional treatment owing to disease progression.

One experiment we conduct to test the anti-cancer effects of a treatment is to draw blood from a man in the lifestyle modification program and add it to a test tube containing cancer cells. We then compare the effect of that serum on the growth of those cells with the effect of serum from a control patient. In Ornish's study group, serum from men in the lifestyle intervention program inhibited the growth of prostate cancer cells *eight times more* than serum from men in the control group!

These same patients were brought back for a follow-up after another year. Of 49 control subjects—men who weren't in the lifestyle intervention program—13 had undergone conventional prostate cancer therapy by that point. Of the 43 men who were exercising, meditating, eating a low-fat diet composed mostly of vegetables, fruit, and whole grains, and participating in a support group, only 2 needed mainstream treatment by the 2-year mark. Remarkable findings, and consistent with my patients at Columbia University. If we could get this kind of result from a drug without any adverse side effects, you can bet we'd be giving it to every man.

Test-tube studies by this group found that exercise and other lifestyle changes impact prostate cancer cells and normal cells in ways that help explain their effect on progression:

- Exercise affects the expression of cancer-modulating genes in the prostate gland, particularly in early-stage cancer.

- Comprehensive lifestyle changes affect *telomeres*, bits of DNA that sit at each end of a cell's chromosomes. Telomeres protect the cell against premature death and cancerous changes. Lifestyle modification affects the speed with which telomeres shorten and eventually disappear, leaving the cell vulnerable to cancerous transformation. An enzyme called telomerase helps to maintain and rebuild telomeres. Researchers can use telomerase activity as a measurement of disease risk, progression, and death in prostate cancer and in other cancers as well. In 24 men with low-risk prostate cancer, Dr. Ornish's group found that 3 months on the lifestyle intervention program significantly increased telomerase activity.

You might be fine with starting a workout program but not so fine with the idea of meditation, yoga, or sitting down with other men in a support group; but the fact is that all of these interventions go together. They're more effective than any one intervention by itself. When it comes to cancer control, a more focused effort to defuse stress and its physical effects is just as important as regular workouts.

The Role of Stress Reduction in Preventing Cancer Growth and Spread

A substantial body of research supports a role for behavioral and social factors in the development and progression of cancer. Stress, chronic depression, and lack of social support increase risk. So does suppressing negative emotions or living in an unremedied state of hopelessness. We've seen this in animal experiments, where cancer growth can be accelerated by creating stressful situations; and we've seen it in studies of human cancer risk and levels of stress, depression, isolation, and social support.

The *stress response* is a complex series of physiological changes in the body, triggered by the response of the brain to whatever situation is causing stress. When we are on high alert, our brains signal fight-or-flight hormonal responses that increase blood pressure, respiratory rate, and heart rate. Stress also increases alertness and suppresses appetite and sex drive. (In an emergency, the last thing you need to think about is what to have for dinner or whether you're in the mood for love.) The main hormones that modulate these changes are called catecholamines. When longer-term stresses are at hand, the brain signals the adrenal glands to produce more of a hormone called cortisol, which alters blood sugar and energy levels.

Having a strong stress response is a good thing in the face of grave danger. The response is designed to create energy, strength, and focus when fighting or fleeing is necessary. In the days when we had to hunt and gather to nourish ourselves, the stress of being hungry made us better, more alert hunters and gatherers.

In modern life, we live with an unprecedented level of slow-burning stress—stress that never really resolves. Levels of stress hormones stay chronically elevated. Chronically elevated cortisol has been linked with abdominal weight gain, lowered immunity, and chronic fatigue. Cellular repair and replacement becomes a low priority when the body is convinced that disaster lurks around every corner. This creates a situation at the cellular level where organs can be damaged and cancer formation and progression become more likely.

Chronic stress appears to impair the feedback system that signals the body to curtail inflammation. This feedback system is supposed to reduce production of stress hormones once they reach a certain level, but when stress is chronic, the system may be overridden. This is one effect of stress that can be counteracted successfully with participation in a support group.

Both frequent, short-term stress and longer-lasting stress raise the risk of heart attack by creating excess tension in blood vessel walls, making them more vulnerable to damage. The immune system then mounts an effort to repair artery walls, but in a body that is already prone to inflammation (due to the factors described in Chapter 2, the response is often excessive.

Chronic stress amplifies free radical production. This psychologically mediated oxidation may directly impact DNA in ways that increase cancer risk. Chronic stress also creates a situation where free radicals are more likely to attack fats floating in the bloodstream, which further increases damage to the arteries and can lead to heart disease. Research also shows that stress significantly decreases the function of *natural killer* cells, immune cells that are our natural allies against cancer.

How to Defuse Stress Effectively

In the Ornish studies, men participated in a program that involved yoga, meditation, breathing exercises, relaxation, guided imagery, and support groups led by trained therapists. These interventions reduce blood pressure, heart rate, and respiratory rate; bring a sense of relaxed well-being; reduce levels of circulating stress hormones; and increase *parasympathetic tone* (activity in the part of the nervous system that opposes the *sympathetic*, fight-or-flight system and becomes better at overriding the sympathetic nervous system when we regularly engage in stress reduction practices).

Personally, I'm a big fan of yoga. This ancient Asian Indian practice—as it's practiced in the West—includes a series of poses designed to stretch and strengthen the body (hatha yoga), performed in a meditative frame of mind, along with deep, measured breathing. This practice is a great combination of strength building, deep breathing (which quiets the sympathetic nervous system and calms the mind), meditation, and stretching.

If you are already involved in a yoga practice, you're moving in the right direction. Just be sure your teacher is incorporating the meditative and breathwork elements of the practice, not just treating the postures as part of a vigorous workout. An overachiever mind-set can easily creep in when the poses are seen as simple physical exercises, and that goes against the whole notion of using yoga as a stress reducer.

If this sounds like something you wouldn't touch with a ten-foot pole, pause before making up your mind. You don't have to be flexible to do yoga, although a peek at a yoga magazine or a yoga class might lead you to think that yoga is for 23-year-olds with taut bodies and a natural ability to contort themselves into pretzel-like shapes. Yoga can be practiced by people of all ages, sizes, and body types; all you need to do is find a class that's right for your level of flexibility and fitness. Don't assume because one class was too strenuous—or demanded a level of flexibility you have only dreamed of—that yoga's not for you. Try a few different teachers and a few different styles of yoga.

Yoga Styles: A Primer

Understanding the differences among styles of practice will help you choose a class that is both challenging and within your abilities. Here are a few types of classes you might see advertised at studios and gyms:

Flow yoga/"power yoga"/vinyasa yoga: Usually a mixed bag that depends on the teacher's preferred style(s). Most classes of this type are based on ashtanga yoga, a rigorous practice of a set series of challenging postures. Standing poses are linked with specific movements called sun salutations. Flow/vinyasa yoga tends not to hold poses for very long and can be challenging in terms of endurance and strength. This is a good type of yoga for men who like a hard workout.

Iyengar yoga: Physically rigorous, involving poses held for long periods of time. Strong emphasis is placed on proper alignment. Props like blocks and straps are often used to allow every student to attain the right alignment in each pose.

Anusara yoga: A blend of Iyengar and a few more modern alignment principles. Like Iyengar, it's rigorous and challenging.

Bikram yoga: A set series of postures performed in a very hot room (sometimes as hot as 100 degrees). Okay for fit men in decent health, but not recommended for those who are being treated for cancer or are not very fit.

Restorative yoga: Performed primarily in a back-lying position using props like blankets, blocks, and straps to hold the body in place. This is a great alternative for men who need lots of stress reduction and not much else—for example, men who are being treated for prostate cancer or are generally not feeling their best.

Hatha (or just plain) yoga: A mixed bag of styles—some take a more vigorous approach while others incorporate lots of rest and restoration. Watch a new teacher's class once or just try it out without pushing beyond your comfort zone to decide whether his or her style works for you.

Men who would rather avoid yoga can try tai chi or chi kung, moving meditative practices from the Far East. Whether you choose yoga, tai chi, or chi kung, there is some initial expense for classes, but once you learn the ropes, you can create your own practice to do at home for free. Even without a movement component, simple or guided meditation, deep breathing, and progressive relaxation will help reduce stress levels. You'll just have to put in extra time and effort with your exercise program.

Meditation, progressive relaxation, and visualization are all effective tools for defusing stress. You can practice one or more of these techniques daily or even twice a day. They can also be used in moments of particular stress: when getting ready for an important meeting, preparing for a difficult conversation, or waiting for results of a medical test. Develop a whole spectrum of stress-coping skills to draw upon in a routine way and when times get tough. The less time overall you spend in a state of anxiety and stress, the stronger your body will be in its resistance to cancer growth and spread.

Meditation can be as simple as sitting in a chair or on a cushion on the floor and paying attention to your breath. Close your eyes, relax your forehead, sit up straight and tall, and make your breaths smooth and regular. When thoughts come, observe them—"Oh, I'm having that thought right now"—and let them go. Sit in this way for 5 to 10 minutes twice a day. (Use a timer so that you don't need to open your eyes to check the clock.) If you like the idea of guided meditation, purchase an audio guide; many can be found online or in stores. Soothing music might also help you relax into your happy place.

Deep breathing. Sit or lie down. Exhale fully, hollowing your belly. Then inhale for a count of 6 to 8; take the same amount of time to exhale. Let chest, ribs, abdomen, and back move with the breath. Repeat 20 to 30 times. In stressful situations, bring back this breathing style to reduce fight-or-flight reactions.

Progressive relaxation. Tense individual muscle groups for 5 to 10 seconds, then release. Doing this in a lying-down position has the best tension-releasing effect. For example, tense the feet and legs, then release; tense the buttocks and hips, then release; tense the abdomen and lower back, then release; and so on up the body until you reach the scalp and face.

Visualization. Picture yourself in a place that is safe, calming, and relaxing. This might be a vacation spot you love or a place you've seen only in pictures.

Finally, don't underestimate the value of laughter in reducing stress and improving the general biochemical condition of your body. Whatever it takes—a funny movie, a board game, a funny blog—find something to give you a good bout of belly laughter at least once a day.

Finding a Support Group

Support groups are another essential ingredient in a stress reduction program for men dealing with prostate cancer or PIN. Do your best to find a group that meets in person with a trained therapist. Your medical team may be able to direct you to a group near you. Us TOO, an advocacy organization that maintains a great online information center for prostate cancer patients, has a database of hundreds of prostate cancer support groups across the

United States, with directions for how to contact these groups: http://www.ustoo.org/Chapter_NearYou. asp?country1=United%20States. Other resources for finding support groups include:

- http://www.cancerfacts.com, which offers a list of support groups in various parts of the United States

- http://www.malecare.com, the site of Malecare, Inc., an organization that supports men fighting cancer

- http://www.cancer.org, the site of the American Cancer Society's Man to Man program (look for "In Your Area")

- http://www.naspcc.com, the site of the National Alliance of State Prostate Cancer Coalitions

- http://www.prostatecancer.ca/pccn.aspx, the site of the Prostate Cancer Canada Network

Exercise for Chemoprevention

Research shows that exercise does make a difference in cancer risk, even if it isn't coupled with the other interventions described in this chapter. Between 1998 and 2008, Harvard University researchers enrolled just under 3,000 men with non-metastatic prostate cancer in the Health Professionals Follow-Up Study. Men who walked 90 or more minutes a week at a normal to fast pace (or who did the equivalent in terms of physical activity) had a 49 percent lower risk of dying from any cause during the years they were followed. They also had a 61 percent lower risk of dying from prostate cancer. Lowest risk was seen in men who exercised vigorously (faster pace) before and after diagnosis. Whether a man wants to prevent or curb prostate cancer or he has undergone treatment and wants to prevent a recurrence, exercise should be a regular part of his life. Moderate exercise soothes inflammation, improves immune system function, and enhances the body's production of natural antioxidant substances. It keeps muscles strong, promotes cardiovascular health, and helps prevent age-related bone loss.

The big picture of exercise is quite simple: Exercise is a good idea, and doing it every day or almost every day is best. Although a vast variety of systems and modes of exercise are advertised and promoted, an ideal exercise program can be incredibly simple. If you take a brisk walk for a half hour a day and do enough push-ups, sit-ups, and bicep curls to exhaust your muscles 3 days a week, you're doing enough to reduce your risk of developing or dying from prostate cancer. Some men will just enjoy doing more or having a more complex program.

Take care to avoid a "no pain, no gain" mind-set when it comes to exercise for chemoprevention. Overdoing it will end up creating *more* stress, more oxidation, and more tissue damage.

Aim for a half hour to an hour a day of sustained physical activity at a pace that feels comfortable. You should be able to speak complete sentences without gasping for breath while doing cardiovascular exercise. When weight training, perform a single set of 8 to 12 repetitions of each exercise using enough weight so that you're too fatigued to perform another repetition with proper form. A session or two with a personal trainer can help a lot to set you up with a program that's easy to follow. The trainer will teach you proper form and alignment, which will help you to avoid injury. Stretching is important for musculoskeletal health. If you aren't practicing yoga, stretch just after working out, when your muscles are warm. Seek the help of a trainer or take a class if you aren't sure how to stretch safely. One thing to keep in mind is that stretching too fast or too hard can cause injury. Always stretch in a relaxed, gradual way. Take deep breaths and ease into your stretches on the exhalation. Adding more activity to your life in general will help, too: Walk more, bike more, take your car less, and make different choices when it comes to recreation. Replace inactive pastimes, like sitting on the couch watching football on TV, with something active, like hiking or playing catch in the park.

PART IV

OTHER PROSTATIC MISHAPS: BPH AND PROSTATITIS

CHAPTER 11

THE "GROWING PROBLEM": INTEGRATIVE DIAGNOSIS AND TREATMENT OF BENIGN PROSTATIC HYPERPLASIA

Benign prostatic hyperplasia (BPH) strikes American men in epidemic proportions. As much as 90 percent of men ages 70 to 90 and over half of men ages 60 to 70 experience some degree of BPH. Not all of these men will require treatment, but their prostates are bigger than they once were.

Symptoms that merit a checkup and treatment for BPH—and the ruling out of something more serious, like prostate cancer—include:

Frequent or urgent need to urinate

Increased frequency of urination at night (*nocturia*)

Difficulty starting the stream of urine

Weak urine stream

Straining during urination

Stopping and starting while urinating

Dribbling at the end of urination

Not being able to empty the bladder completely

Blood in urine (hematuria)

Bladder or kidney stones or frequent urinary tract infections may also suggest a need for a BPH checkup.

In rare cases, a man's first real sign of BPH is a sudden inability to urinate. This is an emergency and requires a doctor's visit for catheterization. If this happens in the middle of the night, it requires an emergency room visit. Known as acute urinary retention, this condition can also be caused by certain over-the-counter cold and allergy medications.

If this happens, I usually recommend a medication such as an alpha-blocker (Flomax, Rapaflo, or UroXatral) for at least 1 week during catheterization. Although I do think there is a role for herbal therapies in men with BPH and lower urinary tract symptoms, retention means immediate medical therapy. It's not something to fool around with.

On that note:

It is very important to treat BPH promptly and thoroughly. Untreated BPH can cause pressure to build up in the bladder and then in the kidneys, which can cause permanent damage. The end-stage result of untreated BPH could be having to wear a urinary catheter for the rest of your days—or worse, the need for dialysis.

Mild BPH may respond to holistic treatments (such as the herbs saw palmetto and pygeum) alone. If medical treatment is required, rest assured that in recent years treatments for BPH have advanced nearly as much as treatments for prostate cancer. Most are minimally invasive and can be done on an outpatient basis.

Causes of BPH

Simple aging is the main driver of prostate enlargement. As men age, their levels of the protective kind of testosterone fall; levels of dihydrotestosterone (DHT), a type of testosterone that accelerates prostate growth, rise; and levels of estrogens, which promote growth in the prostate, also rise. Blocking DHT production with medications is one way we can shrink the prostate in men with the "growing problem" and reduce the risk of urinary retention.

Family history plays a role here, too. Men whose fathers or brothers have BPH are more likely to have it themselves. I routinely ask patients whether prostate conditions are prevalent in their family, and in my own clinical experience I've found family history to be a common factor. White and black men are more likely to have BPH than men of other ethnicities.

What about diet? The largest investigation to date on the role of diet in causing BPH involved 4,770 men who were free of BPH at the beginning of the study. Researchers from the Fred Hutchinson Cancer Research Center in Seattle, Washington, tracked the men for 7 years, keeping data on their dietary choices. When 876 cases of BPH were diagnosed in this group, the study's authors could look at how their diets differed.

The big surprise was that alcohol consumption seemed protective. Men who consumed two or more alcoholic drinks per day had significantly lower risk of developing BPH than men who drank less. Not surprisingly, consuming four or more servings of vegetables per day was protective, while eating red meat more than once a week raised BPH risk. Higher intake of the micronutrients lycopene, zinc, and vitamin D were associated with a lower risk of BPH.

Since 1995, 14 studies have investigated the clinical relationship between exercise and BPH. No randomized controlled trials have been performed, but very interesting information has come from these studies. Most of them support a clinically significant, independent, strong inverse relationship between development of BPH and exercise. In other words, a man who gets regular exercise seems to cut his risk of BPH. Exercise affects the body in several ways that might explain this relationship: It decreases "fight or flight" nervous system activity in the body and may reduce free radical stress in the prostate gland.

Tests for BPH

If you visit your urologist with complaints of BPH symptoms, you'll undergo a series of tests, including a digital rectal exam and PSA blood test. If there is a significant PSA elevation or the rectal exam reveals a nodule, you will likely need to have a prostate biopsy and/ or rectal ultrasound. You may also be given:

A urinary flow test, where you urinate into a container that is attached to a machine that measures the strength of your urine flow and the amount you can urinate. This flow test may be used to monitor your progress during treatment.

A postvoid residual volume test, which uses ultrasound or a catheter to measure how much urine is left in your bladder after you urinate.

Flexible cystoscopy, where an instrument called a cystoscope is inserted through the urethra to have a look inside the bladder. The area is numbed with a small amount of local anesthetic jelly first. In rare cases, a cystoscopy may lead to a urinary tract infection or worsen an existing infection, so your urologist may choose to give you antibiotics before and after the test. I routinely obtain urine for a culture beforehand to make sure there is no infection before doing the cystoscopy. Cystoscopy usually causes small amounts of blood to show up in the urine following the test, but bleeding can be serious in a very small proportion of men. Mild pain and burning during urination are not unusual following cystoscopy. Fever or bright red blood in urine are signs to head back to your doctor for a follow-up exam.

If these tests don't reveal a problem in the urinary tract or with the prostate (BPH, kidney or bladder stones or infections, prostate or urinary tract cancer, or prostatitis), your doctor might suspect heart failure, diabetes, neurological problems, stroke, or muscle or nerve disorders. A neurological exam or other tests may be called for.

If BPH is the diagnosis, your urologist will make recommendations about what next steps to take. You may be advised simply to make a few changes in your habitual consumption of water, alcohol, and caffeinated beverages and take a saw palmetto supplement; you might get a prescription medication; or you might be told that surgery is your best option for total relief from BPH.

Lifestyle Changes

A few simple shifts that can help control enlarged prostate symptoms:

Don't drink for the last hour or two before bed.

Reduce your intake of caffeinated beverages and alcohol, which can irritate the bladder.

The International Prostate Symptom Score

The American Urological Association has developed a questionnaire to help men determine how bothersome their urinary symptoms are and to periodically monitor the effectiveness of treatment. This questionnaire, which has been adopted worldwide, is known as the international prostate symptom score (IPSS).

Use the following point scale to answer the questions:

0 points means you answered "never" to the question.

1 point means you answered "less than 1 out of 5 times" to the question.

2 points means you answered "less than half of the time" to the question.

3 points means you answered "about half of the time" to the question.

4 points means you answered "more than half of the time" to the question.

5 points means you answered "almost always" to the question.

For example, for question number 1, a man who had the feeling of not completely emptying his bladder less than half the time (but more than 1 out of 5 times) would get 2 points for that question. For question number 4, a man who found it hard to hold his urine less than once out of every times would get 1 point for that question.

Prostate Symptom Score Questions

1. Over the past month, how often have you had the feeling of not completely emptying your bladder after you finished urinating?

2. Over the past month, how often have you had to urinate again less than 2 hours after you finished urinating?

3. Over the past month, how often have you found that you stopped and started again several times when you urinated?

4. Over the past month, how often have you found it hard to hold your urine?

5. Over the past month, how often have you had a weak urine stream?

6. Over the past month, how often have you had to push or strain to begin urination?

7. Over the past month, have you had to get up to urinate during the night? Give a score to the number of times.

0 means you did not get up at all.

1 means you got up 1 time.

2 means you got up 2 times.

3 means you got up 3 times.

4 means you got up 4 times.

5 means you got up 5 times or more.

Total your score.

Your score shows how severe your symptoms are, and the symptom index in this questionnaire may help your doctor develop a treatment plan. Expect to be asked to take this test again once treatment has begun to see how well it is helping your symptoms. Sometimes the questionnaire also includes a quality of life scale.

Compare your total score with the following list.

Score and Severity of Problem

SCORE	SEVERITY
0–7	Mild
8–19	Moderate
20–35	Severe

Men who take diuretics, which are generally used to control high blood pressure, may be able to lower their dosage, switch medications, or take their meds earlier in the day so that nighttime urination isn't as much of a problem.

Set a schedule for urination, so that you make sure to go every 4 to 6 hours. This can help to retrain a bladder that has become irritable because of BPH.

Try double voiding: When you urinate, try to urinate more after you finish the first round.

Become more attentive to your urges to urinate. Go as soon as you first feel the urge. This will help prevent bladder muscles from becoming overstretched, which in turn will help with draining the bladder completely.

If you take antihistamines or decongestants, try taking fewer or weaning yourself off them completely. One side effect of these drugs is a constriction of the band of muscle around the urethra—the one that's designed to hold urine in the bladder until you're ready to urinate.

Exercise. Even mild, short bouts of exercise can help relieve BPH symptoms. Keeping your body warm with activity and with warm clothing also helps relax a tensed-up urinary tract.

Herbs for BPH

When BPH is mild enough that medical treatment isn't needed, herbs can promote better urinary function and shrinkage of an enlarged prostate. Try herbs individually to see which ones help, or try a combination product like ProstaCaid, which includes many of these medicinal herbs. New Chapter makes a product called Prostate 5LX, which contains extracts of saw palmetto, green tea, nettle root, rosemary, and selenium.

Another good combination product, made by Quality of Life Labs, is called ProstaCell. I helped to design this product based on current herbal and nutritional research.

Saw palmetto

Saw palmetto (*Serenoa serrulata*) is a dwarf palm tree that grows in coastal areas of the southeastern United States. The berries of the saw palmetto tree contain natural DHT inhibitors. Since the early 19th century, Western medicine has been intrigued by the positive effects of saw palmetto on men with urinary problems.

Studies have looked closely at the molecular effects of saw palmetto in prostate tissue. It appears to work by interfering with the binding of DHT to prostate tissue by blocking the alpha receptors—the same receptors blocked by commonly used prescription BPH medications.

A look at the research on saw palmetto and BPH can be confusing. A meta-analysis (analysis of data from multiple studies) published in the year 2000 found that saw palmetto was significantly better than a placebo in reducing urinary symptoms and improving sexual performance in men with BPH. Other studies suggest that saw palmetto is just as effective as finasteride, a commonly used drug treatment that has some unsavory side effects.

On the other hand, a meta-analysis in the same medical journal in 2009 found no difference in outcome between men on saw palmetto and men taking placebo pills. In fact, for just about every research study that shows that saw palmetto helps, another seems to show that it doesn't! (This also happens with prescription drugs—sometimes a drug we think will have benefit turns out not to have one in the end.) This could be due to differences in the kind of supplement being used or other factors we haven't considered yet.

What I know from my own clinical experience is that saw palmetto has benefited my patients a great deal. In cases of mild BPH, saw palmetto supplements help reduce symptoms in about 70 percent of the men I recommend it to, and this has prevented many of my patients from needing medication or surgery. Although I can't think of any patient for whom I had to stop recommending this herb because of side effects, there have been reports of gastrointestinal upset, abdominal pain, dizziness, headache, and decreased libido or breast enlargement. These side effects are all reversible with discontinuation of the supplement.

Dosage: 160 mg twice a day.

Pygeum

This herb comes from the bark of an African evergreen that grows to 100 feet or more in height. Research evidence suggests that pygeum reduces BPH symptoms by inhibiting prostate cell proliferation, enhancing apoptosis in BPH tissues, inhibiting the formation of pro-inflammatory eicosanoids, and acting as an antiandrogen. It has diuretic effects and enhances prostatic secretions.

Dosage: 50 mg twice daily or 100 mg once daily.

Nettle root

Nettle root is an herb that has been found to help improve urinary function in men with BPH. It affects the binding of estrogens to a protein called sex hormone–binding globulin (SHBG) in a way that may reduce estrogen's impact on the prostate gland. It also inhibits an enzyme called aromatase, which transforms testosterone into growth-promoting estrogens. Some men find benefit from combining the DHT-reducing actions of pygeum with the estrogen-reducing actions of nettle root.

Dosage: 300 to 600 mg twice a day.

Cernilton

Cernilton is a flower pollen extract manufactured in Sweden by AB Cernelle. In Europe and Scandinavia, Cernilton has been used as a plant medicine for decades. It is commonly administered for prostatitis because of its relaxant effect on urethral smooth muscle, but it has also been reported to slow prostate cell growth in BPH. In one study, 240 men with BPH took either 375 or 750 mg of Cernilton twice a day for 4 years. Overall the changes were significant, with the higher dose seeming to have a more beneficial effect on urine flow, urinary retention, and postvoid residual urine. Cernilton users were less likely to require surgery.

Dosage: 160 mg three times a day, or 375 to 750 mg twice a day, with meals.

Beta-sitosterol

A diet high in plant foods is high in beta-sitosterol, a compound that may help relieve BPH symptoms and aid in reducing high cholesterol. A review of studies on beta-sitosterol in BPH found that when taken as a supplement, this compound improves urinary flow and other symptoms of BPH.

Dosage: 20 mg three times a day.

Medications for BPH

Two classes of drugs, working through different mechanisms, have been approved for treatment of BPH. Proscar (finasteride) and Avodart (dutasteride) work by inhibiting 5-alpha reductase, the enzyme that transforms testosterone into DHT. Hytrin (terazosin), Cardura (doxazosin), Flomax (tamsulosin), and UroXatral (alfuzosin) are alpha-blockers that relax the smooth muscle of the bladder neck to improve urine flow.

5-Alpha Reductase Inhibitors for Prostate Cancer Prevention?

In a 2003 study involving 8,000 men, those who took finasteride for 7 years had a 25 percent reduced risk of a prostate cancer diagnosis compared with a placebo. Unfortunately, a proportion of the men on finasteride who *did* develop prostate cancer had a more aggressive form of cancer than men on the placebo who also developed the disease. Overall, 6.4 percent of cancers diagnosed in finasteride patients were high-grade (Gleason score greater than or equal to 7), while only 5.1 percent of cancers in placebo patients were high-grade. This amounts to a 27 percent greater proportion of high-grade tumors in the finasteride group.

A more recent study (published in 2010) evaluated 7,000 men and found a 23 percent reduction in prostate cancer incidence in men taking dutasteride, another 5-alpha reductase inhibitor. This study showed a much smaller trend toward higher-grade disease in men taking medication. The study's authors concluded that the drug's reduction of prostate volume may contribute to a better chance of finding high-grade cancer when a biopsy is performed. In other words, they believe that the drug

5-Alpha Reductase Inhibitors

5-alpha reductase inhibitors will shrink the prostate to some degree, but symptom relief may be slow—it may take 6 months or more to experience the full extent of that relief. Blocking the production of DHT leads to a reduction in prostate size. Typically, with these drugs, there is about a 50 percent reduction in size by about 6 months to 1 year. This reduction in size also results in a lowering of PSA.

does not cause higher-grade cancer but simply makes it more likely to be found within the study period.

Most urologists today are not prescribing Avodart or Proscar for prevention only, despite the reduction in prostate cancer. In fact, the FDA just rejected a request by GlaxoSmithKline to promote Avodart as a cancer preventive therapy. Considerable controversy remains about the upgrading of cancer in patients from the clinical trial who took the medication. The FDA ruled that although 5-alpha reductase inhibitors reduce the development of lower-grade cancers, these are usually not the cancers that lead to mortality. In addition, as noted previously, these medications can cause side effects. Many men are strongly concerned about the drugs' sexual side effects and the possibility of having no semen during orgasm. When I lecture to other urologists and attend seminars, it is the rare urologist in the audience who is offering these medications to patients without symptoms, just for cancer prevention.

However, if a patient has a strong family history of prostate cancer, elevated PSA, and other important risk factors, I might prescribe these medications for prevention. I might also consider these medications for a man with an elevated PSA and a negative biopsy.

These drugs don't work well on men whose symptoms are mild to begin with, and in some men they don't have any real effect on urine flow or other BPH symptoms, even after a year of use. The best relief, in my experience, occurs in men with urinary symptoms and a prostate bigger than 60 grams.

Side effects differ substantially between these two drug classes, since they affect different parts of the genitourinary tract through different mechanisms. Ten percent of men who take 5-alpha reductase inhibitors experience a short-term reduction in sex drive and may experience impotence and reduced semen production. In fact, many men complain that they lose the ability to ejaculate during orgasm.

Men whose partners could get pregnant need to ensure that their partners don't handle their 5-alpha reductase pills, because the drug can be absorbed through the woman's skin. If she becomes pregnant or is pregnant, exposure to these drugs could cause malformations in the baby. As mentioned earlier, these drugs can lower the level of PSA, which means that the test might not catch prostate cancer should it arise. Many academic urologists believe that if you are on Avodart or Proscar for more than 1 year, your "true" PSA is really double the result that comes back while you are on the medication.

Alpha-blockers

Two types of alpha-blockers are used to treat BPH: short-acting and long-acting. Short-acting alpha-blockers relieve symptoms fairly quickly but don't maintain that relief for as long a period. Long-acting alpha-blockers take longer to bring about relief, but that relief lasts for a longer time. Alpha-blockers don't stop the prostate from growing.

Low blood pressure leading to dizziness is a possible side effect of these medications, as is *retrograde ejaculation*—a condition where semen enters the bladder instead of exiting the body through the urethra. This happens from changes in the wideness of the opening that leads to the bladder; when that opening relaxes in response to the drug, semen takes the path of least resistance and flows into the bladder instead of out of the penis. Unless you're trying to conceive a child, retrograde ejaculation isn't a cause for concern; and it is possible to conceive even if you do have this issue (the man urinates into a sterile container after ejaculating; then the sperm are collected, alkalinized, and used for in vitro fertilization).

Combination therapy is a common alternative in medical treatment of BPH. Studies show that using both types of drugs at once achieves better results than using one or the other. In one study, finasteride and doxazosin in combination reduced BPH progression by 67 percent—about twice as much as either drug alone. If a patient of mine has been on herbals and still has moderate to severe symptoms based on IPSS value, combination therapy is probably going to provide him with the fastest relief.

Here's how I typically handle combination therapy: I'll prescribe the alpha-blocker plus 5-alpha reductase inhibitor for at least 3 months. If the man is feeling better, I'll stop the alphablocker and continue the 5-alpha reductase inhibitor (usually Avodart) for longer. As long as the Avodart is working, my experience is that it should be continued for quite a while, sometimes a few years.

Surgeries for BPH

Like surgeries for prostate cancer, surgical procedures used to treat BPH have the potential to cause incontinence and impotence, although this is way less common than in prostate cancer surgery. Some procedures pose a higher risk than others. The better your sexual function before surgery, the better it's likely to be following surgery. See the information on penile rehabilitation on pages 103 to 106 if you would like to be proactive about regaining the best possible sexual function after your operation.

Retrograde ejaculation is another possible result of BPH procedures and can occur in over 90 percent of men who have them. Keep in mind that retrograde ejaculation does not affect your ability to have an erection or an orgasm; you just won't see any semen during ejaculation. This is also known as dry ejaculation.

Transurethral resection of the prostate (TURP)

This is the oldest and most tried-and-true surgical treatment for BPH. It involves the insertion of an instrument called a resectoscope into the urethra. At the end of the scope is a lens and high-powered light source that allows the surgeon to use small cutting tools (inserted through the scope) to remove tissues inside the prostate.

Think for a moment of the prostate as a bagel, with the hole in the middle as the space for the urethra to travel through. What we're doing with TURP is enlarging the hole in the middle of the bagel so that urine can flow easily from the bladder through the penis. The prostate has a rich blood supply, and to prevent bleeding, we use tools that cauterize blood vessels as the surgeon resects the blocking tissue. Once cut away, these tissues are washed into the bladder, which is then drained at the end of the surgery. The capsule of the prostate is left intact.

TURP is a procedure that yields quick results, opening up the urethra and allowing for good urine flow within a few days. Bleeding and infection are potential aftereffects, so most patients will need to stay overnight in the hospital with a catheter and then leave the following day. By then, the catheter has usually been removed.

Incontinence and impotence are very rare with TURP but can occur in 1 to 2 percent of the patients treated with modern-day technology. Repeat surgeries are required in about 15 percent of men. Typically, this procedure maintains good urinary function for at least 10 years. About 90 percent of men who have BPH surgeries have TURP.

Transurethral incision of the prostate (TUIP or TIP)

Another surgical option for men with a small or moderately enlarged prostate is TUIP, which is also performed intraurethrally. Rather than scooping out the tissue of the prostate, the surgeon performing a TUIP cuts small openings into the prostate and the neck of the bladder to allow the urethra to expand. In rare cases, TUIP may cause impotence, but it is less likely to cause retrograde ejaculation than other procedures and can be used in men with smaller-sized glands and in younger men who are concerned about retrograde ejaculation.

Transurethral microwave thermotherapy (TUMT)

This procedure has been in use since the mid-1990s. A device that emits microwaves is inserted into the urethra, and microwaves are used to heat extra prostate tissue to a temperature that destroys it. The tissue then deteriorates and opens up more space for the urethra. TUMT is an outpatient procedure that requires little recovery time, and it relieves all symptoms of BPH except incomplete emptying of the bladder.

Transurethral needle ablation (TUNA)

I do not do TURP at Columbia University Medical Center. Most patients I have seen who have had it tell me they did not find it helpful. Still, it is used in some centers, so I'll give you the basics on it here.

TUNA is a minimally invasive BPH surgery. Instead of a probe, it uses needles that transmit low-level radiofrequencies. Ultrasound is used to pinpoint the areas of the urethra that we want to target, and a heat shield system protects the urethra against any damage from the heat created during the procedure. This outpatient surgery has not yielded any reports of incontinence or impotence. About 60 percent of men who have this surgery can go home without a cathether after TURP.

Green light laser surgery

This outpatient procedure, which is performed under general anesthesia, uses a cystoscope to pass a laser fiber into the urethra and up against the prostate gland. It takes less than 20 minutes; in the majority of cases, there is no significant bleeding. Men with less enlarged prostates are more likely to benefit from this procedure, but some urologists are performing it on patients with very large glands, since the latest laser fibers are able to generate much more energy. Green light laser surgery has gained wide acceptance in urology as a terrific alternative to TURP. At Columbia University Medical Center, I have performed about 100 of these surgeries, and patient satisfaction is nearly 90 percent.

Following the laser procedure, men may experience burning during urination for a few days, and some blood may appear in the urine; this resolves rather quickly. The majority of my patients tell me that their urinary streams are much stronger right after the procedure and that over time they have had less nighttime frequency and urgency. I have not seen any patient develop urinary incontinence from green light laser surgery. No patient has told me that it has affected his sexual function, either.

Open prostatectomy

This surgery may be required by men with very large prostates (more than 150 grams). It requires a hospital stay and general anesthesia. Blood loss can be significant; it's the only BPH surgery that may require a blood transfusion. Widespread use of medical therapies and the adoption of minimally invasive approaches have rendered open prostatectomy for BPH nearly obsolete. It is rarely performed today.

Stents

For men who cannot or do not want to have surgery or take medications, a stent can be inserted to open the urethra. A stent is a tiny cylinder made from metal or plastic. Once it is inserted, tissue grows around it. This is a rarely used option that can cause urinary tract infections or painful urination.

What to Expect following BPH Surgery

Following any inpatient procedure, catheterization is likely. Some men may experience temporary urinary incontinence during the healing process as the bladder returns to normal. Greater urinary urgency and frequency can also arise right after surgery.

Blood or clots will probably appear in the urine of any man who has just undergone BPH surgery, whether inpatient or outpatient. Listen carefully to your doctor's recommendations about how long to rest up following surgery, and don't rush it.

Be gentle when it comes time to empty your bowels; straining can disrupt the healing of the surgery site. Use a stool softener if you need one, and eat plenty of vegetables to keep the bowels moving easily. Drink lots of water, up to 8 cups a day, to flush the bladder and speed healing.

Will Another Surgery Be Needed?

Only about 10 percent of men who undergo BPH surgical procedures end up requiring an additional surgery. In men who have scarring that causes the bladder neck to shrink, another procedure may be necessary to open that pathway again. If scarring affects the urethra and causes it to shrink, a simple stretching procedure done in the urologist's office usually fixes the problem.

Finding Prostate Cancer following BPH Surgery

Although no causal link has been found between BPH and prostate cancer, prostate tissue removed during a TURP is sent to a pathologist to be checked for the presence of cancer. It is rarely found, but if it is, it's not likely to be aggressive or advanced, and you may not need any additional treatment. Consider it a good motivator to start your holistic chemoprevention program, which is beneficial to the health of your prostate and the rest of you.

CHAPTER 12

A PAIN IN THE PROSTATE: INTEGRATIVE DIAGNOSIS AND TREATMENT OF PROSTATITIS

Men between the ages of 25 and 40 who experience pain or burning when urinating or have difficulty urinating can suspect that they're part of the (approximately) 30 percent of men in that age bracket who develop either acute or chronic prostatitis. Other symptoms can include pain or discomfort in the abdomen, groin, lower back, perineum (area between scrotum and rectum), penis, or testicles, especially while sitting. Pain during orgasm is another common symptom.

Prostatitis is a general term that describes an inflammation of the prostate. It can be caused by infection, but treating the infection with antibiotics doesn't always solve the problem. Nonbacterial prostatitis, where no infection is found to explain the symptoms and inflammation, is more common, and its causes are not well understood. The most promising ideas about it have to do with the role of stress in creating muscular spasms around the prostate gland. Spasms like these are best treated not with antibiotics, but with physical therapy and acupuncture. You will read much more about this in later parts of this chapter.

Men with prostatitis can go a long time with symptoms that don't respond to mainstream medical therapies. If pelvic pain has gone on for 3 months or more, it is classified as chronic. Prostatitis diagnoses fall into one of five categories:

- Acute prostatitis, where pain and bacteria are clearly present. Fever and chills may be present as well. Five to ten percent of men with prostatitis have certifiable infections. We treat these with antibiotics.

- Chronic bacterial prostatitis may or may not involve pain, but white blood cells and bacteria are found in samples of prostatic fluid, semen, and/or urine. This diagnosis is relatively rare. Men who get repeat urinary tract infections may also end up with a diagnosis of chronic bacterial prostatitis. Antibiotics may or may not clear up the problem.

- Inflammatory chronic prostatitis along with chronic pelvic pain syndrome (below), represents 95 percent of all cases of prostatitis. No signs of infection are found in inflammatory chronic prostatitis, but we can detect signs that infection-fighting cells are being produced in the prostate and/or bladder. Symptoms don't resolve when we treat the infection; in fact, symptoms can come and go without seeming cause.

- Chronic pelvic pain syndrome (CPPS), where pain is a symptom, but no infection or signs of inflammation are found. Pain syndromes involving the urinary tract or the prostate gland may be classified together as *urological chronic pelvic pain syndromes*. Loss of libido or erectile function is sometimes reported in CPPS.

• Asymptomatic inflammatory prostatitis causes no symptoms, so it is usually found when white blood cells are detected during evaluations for other conditions. Generally, no treatment is necessary.

Chronic pelvic pain syndrome and inflammatory chronic prostatitis have previously been lumped together under the names chronic nonbacterial prostatitis or prostatodynia. Although a distinction is now made between inflammatory and noninflammatory chronic prostatitis, that distinction isn't really useful when it comes to treatment.

Chronic pelvic pain sufferers have high levels of stress and anxiety. It doesn't help when doctors tell them they don't know what causes their suffering and that there's not much they can do besides sit in warm baths and take 5-alpha reductase inhibitors or alphablocker medications like Flomax to try to relax their tensed-up genitourinary systems. Some men with chronic pelvic pain undergo surgeries or take long courses of antibiotics in attempts to rid themselves of this disorder.

Possible Causes of Prostatitis

Bacterial prostatitis can be a result of urinary tract infection. Infected urine may flow backward into prostate ducts. Rectal bacteria can also move into the urethra and eventually infect the prostate gland. This is especially true of men who engage in rectal intercourse.

Men who use or have recently used urinary catheters are at greater risk of developing bacterial prostatitis. So are men who have abnormalities in their urinary tracts. BPH can also raise the risk of painful prostate inflammation.

Rarer causes of prostatitis may include:

Prostatic stones. About 75 percent of middle-aged men have calcified stones in their prostates. These are made up of "backed up" prostate secretions that are blocked by BPH-induced structural changes. Calcified stones may also form in the ejaculatory ducts. Stones may cause no symptoms at all, or they can trigger chronic prostatitis. Unfortunately, lithotripsy—the method we use to break up kidney stones—is not an effective cure here. We can try prostate massage to try to break up the stones, but this is not always effective. When it is, it may be temporary.

Urethral strictures. The urethra becomes partially closed off by fibrotic tissue buildup, caused by infection or trauma. In men with urethral strictures, repeated bladder infections can end up infecting the prostate. In these men, the bladder may eventually become ineffective at draining itself all the way during urination. Untreated urethral stricture can lead to kidney failure, so it's important to address it as soon as it's detected—which is usually through detection of a significant decrease in the power of the urine stream during an evaluation for urinary tract symptoms. Flow rate, X-ray, and cystoscopy are used to locate the stricture. Treatments may include dilation (filiforms or narrow rods are threaded through the urethra to gradually expand the opening) and urethrotomy (an endoscope with a tiny cutting tool on its end is used to cut out fibrotic tissue inside the urethra). Urethrotomy is successful 70 to 80 percent of the time, but if it doesn't work, the last resort is to surgically remove the fibrotic urethral segment. If it's more than 2 centimeters long, we do a skin graft to help ensure that there's plenty of room in the newly refurbished urethra.

Cancer. In rare cases, chronic prostatitis is caused by undetected cancer. Tests to rule out this possibility may be part of your evaluation.

Pelvic floor muscle spasm. I believe that this may be the main cause of symptoms in over 90 percent of CPPS patients. Any man with CPPS should have a pelvic floor examination by someone expert in trigger point/myofascial evaluation as part of his complete urological work-up. If pelvic floor muscle spasm is present, it can be treated successfully through a protocol developed by Drs. David Wise and Rodney Anderson.

According to Drs. Wise and Anderson, the tension that sets the stage for CPPS is an exaggerated form of the natural human instinct to protect the contents of the pelvis. Over time, muscle tension activates several interrelated body systems that produce pain and (possibly) inflammation in the prostate gland. In their book *A Headache in the Pelvis*, 6th ed. (Occidental, Calif.: National Center for Pelvic Pain, 2010), Wise and Anderson write:

> We have identified a group of chronic pelvic pain syndromes that we believe is caused by the overuse of the human instinct to protect the genitals, rectum, and contents of the pelvis from injury or pain by contracting the pelvic muscles. This tendency becomes exaggerated in predisposed individuals and over time results in chronic pelvic pain and dysfunction. The state of chronic constriction creates pain-referring trigger points, reduced blood flow, and an inhospitable environment for the nerves, blood vessels, and structures throughout the pelvic basin. This results in a cycle of tension, anxiety, and pain . . .

Wise and Anderson's book details a rehabilitation program designed to relax short muscles and stretch connective tissue in the pelvis. In this process, men are guided through a method that helps them to stop creating the tension that ends up causing pain. The Wise-Anderson protocol is recommended by Jeannette Potts, MD, director of the Center for Pelvic Pain, Alternative and Medical Urology Services, Case Western Reserve University in Cleveland, Ohio; Ragi Doggweiler, MD, director of neuro-urology and integrative medicine, Division of Urology, University of Tennessee in Knoxville; Bart Gershbein, MD, clinical instructor, Department of Urology, University of California School of Medicine in San Francisco; and many physical therapists and researchers who specialize in or study pelvic pain syndromes.

Other Treatments for Prostatitis

In my own practice, we usually perform some tests initially to guide the course of prostatitis treatment. We do a urethral swab and a urine test to look for bacteria. I also like to check prostatic secretions (obtained via prostate massage) and/or urine collected following prostate massage. In addition, I ask men with post-ejaculatory pain or changes in the appearance of semen to give a semen sample that we then culture to check for infection.

When bacteria are present, antibiotics may or may not fix the problem. If one antibiotic doesn't work, the bacteria present may be resistant to that drug, and another might do the trick. Nonbacterial prostatitis can evolve from bacterial prostatitis, which means that eradicating the offending "bug" may not resolve the symptoms. More involved testing can be performed if antibiotics don't effect a cure.

Some urologists will simply give a broad-spectrum antibiotic to any man who presents with prostatitis rather than do tests to try to figure out whether bacteria are the cause of the man's discomfort. This kind of so-called empiric treatment appears to be as effective as treatment based on extensive testing to determine whether bacteria are present and which bacteria might be causing the infection. If antibiotics don't work, empirical treatment simply moves on to the next mode of treatment to see whether that works better.

If prostatitis is inflammatory rather than infectious, the most likely reality is that the immune system is detecting some kind of enemy agent in the prostate gland. It mounts an attack on that enemy, producing inflammation and pain, but because of dysregulation in the immune system, the body doesn't shut off the inflammation when appropriate.

One study found that men with chronic nonbacterial prostatitis who abstained from sex tended to see big improvements with twice daily masturbation. Of the 18 men enrolled in the study, 78 percent obtained moderate to complete relief!

All the advice given in the chapter on chemopreventive diet and supplements is appropriate for the man with prostatitis. Staying hydrated will help keep the urinary tract flushed out.

Natural Medicine to Fight Chronic Infection and Promote Better Urinary Function

I mentioned the flower pollen remedy Cernilton in the chapter on BPH (page 209). Cernilton has also been studied as a remedy for chronic prostatitis. Research studies of men with chronic prostatitis have demonstrated that Cernilton works significantly better than a placebo to relieve symptoms and improve quality of life.

Men with bacterial prostatitis or repeated urinary tract infections can fortify their immune systems with herbs and other supplements. These supplements will promote immunity against all infectious invaders. Berberine, which is a plant chemical found in goldenseal, barberry, and Oregon grape, is also recommended in my chemoprevention program (see page 177). It has strong antibacterial effects and is known for its ability to block the adhesion of pathogens to body tissues. Cranberry is a well-known natural remedy for urinary tract infection; it also works by reducing bacteria's ability to adhere to body tissues. Use these herbs together or individually as part of an overall immune-boosting program. I have also recommended that my patients take the herbal anti-inflammatory compound Zyflamend—three pills a day—to help control inflammation and oxidation.

Garlic and echinacea help the body fight infection. Although studies on echinacea are equivocal—some show benefits to immune function, others don't—it has been used for this purpose for thousands of years. Garlic's immune system–boosting properties are well supported by research studies.

Diuretic herbs like couchgrass, pipsissewa, watermelon seed, and queen of the meadow may help promote better urinary tract function. Try them as teas or in capsules. Chamomile, valerian, passionflower, cramp bark, dong quai, and Baikal skullcap are sedative and/or antispasmodic herbs that may help relax tensed-up pelvic muscles. Don't use dong quai if you are diabetic, as it can raise blood sugar levels.

Acupuncture for Chronic Pelvic Pain

At the Center for Holistic Urology, staff acupuncturist Jillian Capodice instituted a study of acupuncture treatment for chronic pelvic pain symptoms. Ten men with symptoms that had lasted 6 months or more underwent twice weekly acupuncture sessions for 6 weeks. Questionnaires given before and after the treatment indicated a significantly positive effect of the treatment. No side effects were noted. Another study of 12 men with chronic prostate pain found that 11 had greater than 50 percent improvement in symptoms, based on the National Institutes of Health chronic prostatitis symptom index. Of those 11, 10 had at least a 75 percent improvement in subjective symptoms. Their improvements were maintained for 24 of 52 weeks of follow-up.

Why would acupuncture work for this disorder? Since we're not entirely sure of all the mechanisms involved in creating CPPS, and we're also not sure of all the ways in which acupuncture works, we can't quite say. According to the tenets of traditional Chinese medicine, prostate dysfunction springs from a deficiency or blockage of vital energy (*chi* or *qi*) in that part of the body. Acupuncture is said to restore the flow of this energy to the prostate, allowing the body to heal itself. At the Center for Holistic Urology, it has helped many men cope with their symptoms.

ACKNOWLEDGMENTS

I would like to thank Melissa Lynn Block, whose writing and editorial support helped make this book a reality; Lacy Lynch and her colleagues at Dupree Miller and Associates; and the stellar editorial staff at Rodale, especially the patient and professional Marie Crousillat.

Also, I wish to thank my parents, Gary and Rochelle Katz, and my wife Jennifer for their love and support. Love and appreciation to my son Alex, who is going through his own battle with cancer; his strength and courage have been an incredble inspiration to me in my own work with patients. The loyalty and support of Alex's two brothers, Jared and Jesse, have been equally inspiring.

Thanks also to Dr. Mitchell Benson and the entire urology staff at Columbia, and to my longtime secretary, Mona Hanoman, my terrific nurse Kerry Cuccia, and my co-host on my radio show, Katz's Corner, Dr. Philippa Cheetham.

REFERENCES

Chapter One: Your Prostate: A User's Guide

Altekruse SF, Kosary CL, Krapcho M, et al. (eds.), *SEER Cancer Statistics Review, 1975-2007*. National Cancer Institute, Bethesda, MD. http://seer.cancer.gov/csr/1975-2007.

Dennis LK, Dawson DV, Resnick MI, "Vasectomy and the risk of prostate cancer: a meta-analysis examining vasectomy status, age at vasectomy and time since vasectomy," *Prostate Cancer Prostatic Diseases* 5, no. 3 (2002):193–203.

Harding, Ann, "Heart deaths, suicides linked to prostate cancer diagnosis," *CNN Health*, February 2, 2010. http://articles.cnn. com/2010-02-02/health/suicide.heart.deaths_1_prostate-cancer-cancer-patients-national-cancer-institute?_s=PM:HEALTH (accessed February 15, 2011).

Chapter Two: Understanding Prostate Cancer (and Cancer in General)

American Cancer Society, *Cancer Facts and Figures 2010*. Atlanta, GA: American Cancer Society, 2010.

Basha R, Baker CH, Sankpal UT, et al., "Therapeutic applications of NSAIDs in cancer: special emphasis on tolfenamic acid," *Front Biosci* 3 (School Edition) (January, 2011): 797–805.

Chow W-H, Dong LM, and Devesa SS, "Epidemiology and risk factors for kidney cancer," *Nature Reviews Urology* 7, no. 5 (2010): 245–257.

Daniels NA, Nielson CM, Hoffman AR, et al., "Sex hormones and the risk of incident prostate cancer," *Urology* 76, no. 5 (November 2010):1034–40.

Harris RE, Beebe-Donk J, Doss H, et al., "Aspirin, ibuprofen and other non-steroidal anti-inflammatory drugs in cancer prevention: a critical review of non-selective COX-2 blockade (review)," *Oncol Rep* 13, no. 4 (April 2005): 559–83.

Iguchi T, Wang CY, Delongchamps NB, et al., "Occult prostate cancer affects the results of case-control studies due to verification bias," *Anticancer Research* 28, no. 5B (2008): 3007–10.

Mahmud SM, Franco EL, Turner D et al., "Use of non-steroidal anti-inflammatory drugs and prostate cancer risk: a population-based, nested cause-control study," *PLOS One* 28, no. 6 (January 2011): e16412.

Pereg D, Lishner M, "Non-steroidal anti-inflammatory drugs for the prevention and treatment of cancer," *J Intern Med* 258, no. 2 (August 2005):115–23.

Racaniello, Vincent. "The amazing HeLa cells of Henrietta Lacks," *Virology Blog*, February 9, 2009, http://www.virology.ws/2009/02/09/the-amazing-hela-cells-of-henrietta-lacks/. (Accessed December 8, 2010).

Severi G, Morris HA, MacInnis RI, et al., "Circulating steroid hormones and the risk of prostate cancer," *Cancer Epidemiol Biomarkers Prev* 15, no.1 (January 2006):86–91.

Chapter Three: Understanding Integrative Medicine and Its Scientific Foundations

Center for Disease Control and Prevention. *National Health Interview Survey*. Atlanta, GA: Center for Disease Control and Prevention. http://www.cdc.gov/nchs/data/nhis/earlyrelease/earlyrelease201106.pdf. (Accessed April 12, 2011).

Chapter Four: The Truth About Prostate Cancer Screening and Diagnosis: What Tests are Really Needed and Why

Andriole GL, Crawford ED, Grubb RL 3rd, et al., "Mortality results from a randomized prostate-cancer screening trial," *N Engl J Med* 360, no. 13 (March 2009): 1310–9. Epub 2009, Mar 18.

Bankhead C, "ACS Pushes for Shared Decisions for Prostate Screening," *MedPage Today*, http://www.medpagetoday.com/Oncology/ProstateCancer/18799. (Accessed February 12 2011).

Bastian PJ, Carter BH, Bjartell A, Seitz M, Stanislaus P, Montorsi F, Stief CG, Schröder F, "Insignificant prostate cancer and active surveillance: from definition to clinical implications," *Eur Urol* 55, no. 6 (June 2009): 1321–30.

Carlsson S, Aus G, Bergdahl S, Khatami A, Lodding P, Stranne J, Hugosson J, "The excess burden of side-effects from treatment in men allocated to screening for prostate cancer. The Göteborg randomised population-based prostate cancer screening trial," *Eur J Cancer* 47, no. 4 (March 2011): 545–53. Epub: November 2010.

Hugosson J, Carlsson S, Aus G, Bergdahl S, Khatami A, Lodding P, Pihl CG, Stranne J, Holmberg E, Lilja H, "Mortality results from the Göteborg randomised population-based prostate-cancer screening trial," Lancet Oncol. 11, no. 8 (August 2010): 725–32. Epub: July 2010.

Welch HG, Albertson PC, "Prostate cancer diagnosis and treatment after the introduction of prostate-specific antigen screening, 1986-2005," *J Nat Canc Inst* 101, no. 19 (2009): 1325–29.

Wolf AMD, et al., "American Cancer Society guideline for the early detection of prostate cancer, updated 2010," *CA Cancer J Clin* 60 (2010): epub.

Chapter Five: Staging Tests for Prostate Cancer

[NO REFERENCES FOR THIS CHAPTER]

Chapter Six: Not Your Father's Prostate Cancer Treatments: The Truth about Mainstream Medical Therapy for Prostate Cancer

Cheetham P, Truesdale M, Chaudhury S, et al., "Long-term cancer-specific and overall survival for men followed more than 10 years after primary and salvage cryoablation of the prostate," *J Endourol* 24, no. 7 (July 2010): 1123–9.

Glickman L, Godoy G, Lepor H, "Changes in continence and erectile function between 2 and 4 years after radical prostatectomy," *J Urol.* 181, no. 2 (February 2009): 731–5. Epub: December 2008.

Hu JC, "Comparative effectiveness of minimally invasive vs. open radical prostatectomy," *JAMA* 302 (2009): 1557–1564.

Mottet N, Bellemunt J, Bolla M, et al., "EAU Guidelines on Prostate Cancers. Part II: Treatment of Advanced, Relapsing, and Castration-Resistant Prostate Cancer," *Eur Urol.* 59, no. 4 (April 2011): 572–83.

Mulhall JP, and Morgentaler A, "Penile rehabilitation should become the norm for radical prostatectomy patients," *J Sex Med* 4 (2007): 538–543.

UCSF Medical Center, "Active Surveillance for Prostate Cancer," interview with Dr. Peter Carroll, http://www.ucsfhealth.org/education/active_surveillance_for_prostate_cancer/. (Accessed March 12 2011).

No authors listed, "Goodbye watchful waiting. Hello active surveillance." www.cpn.org/arch_0025_watchful.htm. Accessed 3-12-11.

Parker-Pope, Tara, "On sex after prostate surgery, confusing data," *New York Times*, January 15, 2008, www.nytimes.com/2008/01/15/health/15well.html?_r=. (Accessed March 17 2011).

Walsh PC, "Radical prostatectomy for localized prostate cancer provides durable cancer control with excellent quality of life: a structured debate," *J Urol* 163, no. 6 (2000): 1802–7.

Walsh PC, Marschke P, Ricker D, Burnett AL, "Patient-reported urinary continence and sexual function after anatomic radical prostatectomy," *Urology* 55, no. 1 (2000): 58–61.

Wu JN, Dall'Era MA, "Active surveillance for localized prostate cancer— current practices and recommendations," *ScientificWorldJournal* 10, (December 2010): 2352–61.

Chapter Seven: Rising PSA After Treatment

Dorff TB, Flaig TW, Tangen CM, et al., "Adjuvant androgen deprivation for high-risk prostate cancer after radical prostatectomy: SWOG S9921 Study," *J Clin Oncol* 29, no. 15 (May 2011): 2040–5.

Finley DS, Belldegrun AS, "Salvage cryotherapy for radiation-recurrent prostate cancer: outcomes and complications," *Curr Urol Rep* 12, no. 3 (June 2011): 209–15.

Geinitz H, Riegel MG, Thamm R, et al., "Outcome after conformal salvage radiotherapy in patients with rising prostate-specific antigen levels after radical prostatectomy," *Int J Radiat Oncol Biol Phys* (April 2011) http:// www.sciencedirect.com/science/article/pii/S0360301611003774.

Halverson S, Schipper M, Blas K, et al., "The Cancer of the Prostate Risk Assessment (CAPRA) in patients treated with external beam radiation therapy: evaluation and optimization in patients at higher risk of relapse," *Radiother Oncol* (June 2011). http://www.thegreenjournal. com/article/S0167-8140(11)00304-5/abstract.

Hoffman KE, Nguyen PL, Chen MH, et al., "Recommendations for post-prostatectomy radiation therapy in the United States before and after the presentation of randomized trials," *J Urol* 185, no. 1 (January 2011): 116–20.

Huang WC, Lee CL, Eastham JA, "Locally ablative therapies for primary radiation failures: a review and critical assessment of efficacy," *Curr Urol Rep* 8, no. 3 (May 2007): 217–23.

Nielsen ME, Trock BJ, Walsh PC, "Salvage or adjuvant radiation therapy: counseling patients on the benefits," *J Natl Compr Canc Netw* 8, no. 2 (February 2010): 228–37.

Nilsson S, Norlen BJ, Widmark A, "A systematic overview of radiation therapy effects in prostate cancer," *Acta Oncol* 43, no. 4 (2004): 316–81.

Roberts WB, Han M, "Clinical significance and treatment of biochemical recurrence after definitive therapy for localized prostate cancer," *Surg Oncol* 18, no. 3 (September 2009): 268–74.

Showalter TN, Foley KA, Jutkowitz E, et al., "Costs of early adjuvant radiation therapy after radical prostatectomy: a decision analysis," *Ann Oncol* 22, no. 6 (June 2011). http://annonc.oxfordjournals.org/content/early/2011/06/08/annonc.mdr281.long.

Stenmark MH, Blas K, Halverson S, et al., "Continued benefit to androgen deprivation therapy for prostate cancer patients treated with dose-escalated radiation therapy across multiple definitions of high-risk disease," *Int J Radiat Oncol Bio Phys* (June 2011). http://www.sciencedirect.com/science/article/pii/S036030161100558X.

Thoms J, Goda JS, Zlotta AR, et al., "Neoadjuvant radiotherapy for locally advanced and high-risk prostate cancer," *Nat Rev Clin Oncol* 8, no. 2 (February 2011): 107–13.

Tzou K, Tan WW, Buskirk S, "Treatment of men with rising prostate-specific antigen levels following radical prostatectomy," *Expert Rev Anticancer Ther* 11, no. 1 (January 2011): 125–36.

Chapter Eight: The Prostate Cancer Diet

Adhami VM, Khan N, Mukhtar H, "Cancer chemoprevention by pomegranate: laboratory and clinical evidence," *Nutr Cancer* 61, no. 6 (2009): 811–5.

Astorg P, "Dietary N-6 and N-3 polyunsaturated fatty acids and prostate cancer risk: a review of epidemiological and experimental evidence," *Cancer Causes Control* 15, no. 4 (May 2004): 367–86.

Cavazos DA, Price RS, Apte SS, Degraffenried LA, "Docosahexaenoic acid selectively induces human prostate cancer cell sensitivity to oxidative stress through modulation of NF-∞B," *Prostate* (February 2011).

Cavell BE, Syed A, Donlevy A, et al., "Anti-angiogenic effects of dietary isothiocyanates: mechanisms of action and implications for human health," *Biochem Pharmacol* 81, no. 3 (February 2011): 327–36.

Chavarro JE, Stampfer MJ, Hall MN, Sesso HD, Ma J, "A 22-y prospective study of fish intake in relation to prostate cancer incidence and mortality," *Am J Clin Nutr* 88, no. 5 (November 2008): 1297–303.

DeMark-Wahnefried P, Polascik TJ, George SL, et al., "Flaxseed supplementation (not dietary fat restriction) reduces prostate cancer proliferation rates in men presurgery," *Canc Epidem Biom Prev* 17 (December 2008): 3577.

Gupta SC, Kannappan R, Reuter S, et al., "Chemosensitization of tumors by resveratrol," *Ann NY Acad Sci* 1215 (January 2011): 150–60.

Heber D, "Multitargeted therapy of cancer by elagitannins," *Cancer Lett* 269, no. 2 (October 2008): 262–8.

Hebert JR, Hurley TG, Olendzki BC, et al., "Nutritional and socioeconomic factors in relation to prostate cancer mortality: a cross-national study," *J Natl Cancer Inst* 90, no. 21 (November 1998): 1637–47.

Higdon JV, Delage B, Williams DE, "Cruciferous vegetables and human cancer risk: epidemiologic evidence and mechanistic basis," *Pharmacol Res* 55, no 3 (March 2007): 224–36.

Hossain A, Sehbai A, Abraham R, et al, "Cancer health disparities among Indian and Pakistani immigrants in the United States: a surveillance, epidemiology and results-based study from 1988 to 2003," *Cancer* 113 (2008): 1423–30.

Kurahashi N, Iwsaki M, Inoue M, et al., "Plasma isoflavones and subsequent risk of prostate carcinoma in a nested case-control study: The Japan Public Health Center," *J Clin Oncol* 26, no. 36 (December 2008): 5923–9.

Kurahashi N, Iwaski M, Sasazuki S, "Soy product and isoflavone consumption in relation to prostate cancer in Japanese men," *Cancer Epidemiol Biomarkers Prev* 16, no. 3 (March 2007): 538–45.

Lucia MS, "Inflammation as a target for prostate cancer chemoprevention: pathological and laboratory rationale," *Urol Oncol* (March 2011).

MacLean MA, Scott BE, Deziel BA, et al., "North American cranberry (*Vaccinum macrocarpon*) stimulates apoptotic pathways in DU145 human prostate cancer cells in vitro," *Nutr Cancer* 63, no. 1 (January 2011): 109–20.

Moriarty RM, Naithani R, Surve B, et al., "Organosulfur componds in cancer chemoprevention," *Mini Rev Med Chem* 17, no. 8 (August 2007): 827–38.

Nelsom MA, "Inhibition of lipoxygenase activity: implications for the treatment and chemoprevention of prostate cancer," *Cancer Biology & Therapy* 6, no. 2 (February 2007): 237.

Nelson WG, DeMarzo AM, DeWeese TL, "The role of inflammation in the pathogenesis of prostate cancer," *J Urol* 172 no. 5 pt. 2 (November 2004): S6–11; discussion S11–2.

Nelson WG, DeWeese TL, DeMarzo AM, "The diet, prostate inflammation, and the development of prostate cancer," *Cancer and Metastasis Reviews* 21, no. 1: 3–16.

Pew Social Trends Staff, "Eating more, enjoying less," *Pew Research Center*, April 19, 2006. http://pewsocialtrends.org/2006/04/19/eating-more-enjoying-less// (Accessed April 8 2011).

Quinn M, Babb P, "Patterns and trends in prostate cancer incidence, survival, prevalence and mortality. Part I: international comparison," *Int J Cancer (Predictive Oncology)* 85, (2000): 60–67.

Reese AC, Fradet V, Witte JS, "Omega-3 fatty acids, genetic variants in COX-2 and prostate cancer," *J Nutrigenet Nutrigenomics* 2, no. 3 (2009): 149–58. Epub: September 2009.

Schumacher MC, Laven B, Petersson F, Cederholm T, Onelöv E, Ekman P, Brendler C, "A comparative study of tissue ∞-6 and ∞-3 polyunsaturated fatty acids (PUFA) in benign and malignant pathologic stage pT2a radical prostatectomy specimens," Urol Oncol (March 2011).

Sengupta A, Ghosh S, Bhattacharjee S, "Allium vegetables in cancer prevention: an overview," Asia Pac J Cancer Prev 5, no. 3 (July-September 2004): 237–45.

Szymanski KM, Wheeler DC, Mucci LA, "Fish consumption and prostate cancer risk: a review and meta-analysis," Am J Clin Nutr 92, no. 5 (November 2010): 1223–33. Epub: September 2010.

Williams CD, Whitley BM, Hoyo C, et al., "A high ratio of dietary n-6/n-3 polyunsaturated fatty acids is associated with increased risk of prostate cancer," Nutr Res 31, no. 1 (January 2011): 1–8

Wang W, Bergh A, Damber J-E, "Cyclooxygenase-2 expression correlates with local chronic inflammation and tumor neovascularization in human prostate cancer," Clin Cancer Res 11, no. 9 (May 2005): 3250–6.

Chapter Nine: Much More Than Roots, Leaves, and Berries: The Center for Holistic Urology's Herbal and Nutritional Supplement Recommendations

Adhami VM, Khan N, Mukhtar H, "Cancer chemoprevention by pomegranate: laboratory and clinical evidence," Nutr Cancer 61, no. 6 (2009): 811–5.

Bemis DL, Capodice JL, Desai M, Katz AE, Buttyan R, "Beta-carboline alkaloid-enriched extract from the amazonian rain forest tree pao pereira suppresses prostate cancer cells," J Soc Integr Oncol 7, no. 2 (Spring 2009): 59–65.

Bemis DL, Capodice JL, Gorroochurn P, Katz AE, Buttyan R, "Anti-prostate cancer activity of a beta-carboline alkaloid enriched extract from Rauwolfia vomitoria," Int J Oncol 29, no. 5 (November 2006): 1065–73.

Brasky TM, Velicer CM, Kristal AR, et al., "Non-steroidal anti-inflammatory drugs and prostate cancer risk in the VITamins And Lifestyle (VITAL) cohort," Cancer Epidemiol Biomarkers Prev 19, no. 12 (December 2010): 3185–8. Epub: October 2010.

Capodice JL, Gorroochurn P, Cammack AS, Eric G, McKiernan JM, Benson MC, Stone BA, Katz AE, "Zyflamend in men with high-grade prostatic intraepithelial neoplasia: results of a phase I clinical trial," J Soc Integr Oncol 7, no. 2 (Spring 2009): 43–51.

Cavazos DA, Price RS, Apte SS, et al., "Docosahexaenoic acid selectively induces human prostate cancer cell sensitivity to oxidative stress through modulation of NF-kB," *Prostate 2011.*

Dotan N, Wasser SP, Mahajna J., "The Culinary-Medicinal Mushroom Coprinus comatus as a Natural Antiandrogenic Modulator," *Integr Cancer Ther* (December 2010).

Gasmi J, Sanderson JT, "Growth Inhibitory, Antiandrogenic, and Pro-apoptotic Effects of Punicic Acid in LNCaP Human Prostate Cancer Cells," *J Agric Food Chem* (November 2010)

Grant WB, "The roles of ultraviolet-B irradiance, vitamin D, apolipoprotein E4 and diet in the risk of prostate cancer," *Cancer Causes Control* 22, no. 1 (January 2011): 157–8.

Lowe JF, Frazee LA, "Update on prostate cancer chemoprevention," *Pharmacotherapy* 26, no. 3 (March 2006): 353–9.

Newsom-Davis TE, Kenny LM, Ngan S, "The promiscuous receptor," *BJU Int* (November 2009): 1204–7.

Pathak SK, Sharma RA, Steward WP, Mellon JK, Griffiths TR, Gescher AJ, "Oxidative stress and cyclooxygenase activity in prostate carcinogenesis: targets for chemopreventive strategies," *Eur J Cancer* 41, no. 1 (January 2005): 61–70.

Rafailov S, Cammack S, Stone BA, Katz AE, "The role of Zyflamend, an herbal anti-inflammatory, as a potential chemopreventive agent against prostate cancer: a case report," *Integr Cancer Ther* 6, no. 1 (March 2007): 74–6.

Sandur SK, Ahn KS, Ichikawa H, et al., "Zyflamend, a polyherbal preparation, inhibits invasion, suppresses osteoclastogenesis, and potentiates apoptosis through down-regulation of NF-kappa B activation and NF-kappa B-regulated gene products," *Nutr Cancer* 57, no. 1 (2007): 78–87.

Schmid HP, Engeler DS, Pummer K, et al., "Prevention of prostate cancer: more questions than data," *Recent Results Cancer Res* 174 (2007): 101–7.

Sliva D, "Ganoderma lucidum (Reishi) in cancer treatment," *Integr Cancer Ther* 2, no. 4 (December 2003): 358–64.

Wei MY, Giovannucci EL, "Vitamin D and multiple health outcomes in the Harvard cohort," *Mol Nutr Food Res* 54, no. 8 (August 2010): 1114–26.

Williams CD, Whitley BM, Grant DJ, et al., "A high ration of dietary n-6/n-3 polyunsaturated fatty acids is associated with increased risk of prostate cancer," *Nutr Res* 31, no. 1 (January 2011): 1–8.

Weng CJ, Yen GC, "The in vitro and in vivo experimental evidences disclose the chemopreventive effects of Ganoderma lucidum on cancer invasion and metastasis," *Clin Exp Metastasis* 27, no. 5 (May 2010): 361–9. Epub: May 2010.

Yan J, Katz AE, "ProstaCaid induces G2/M cell cycle arrest and apoptosis in human and mouse androgen-dependent and-independent prostate cancer cells," *Integr Cancer Ther* 9, no. 2 (June 2010): 186–96.

Yang P, Cartwright C, Chan D, et al., "Zyflamend-mediated inhibition of human prostate cancer PC3 cell proliferation: effects on 12-LOX and Rb protein phosphorylation," *Cancer Biology & Therapy* 6, no. 2 (February 2007): 228–236.

Zaidman BZ, Wasser SP, Nevo E, Mahajna J, "Coprinus comatus and Ganoderma lucidum interfere with androgen receptor function in LNCaP prostate cancer cells," *Mol Biol Rep* 35, no. 2 (June 2008): 107–17. Epub: March 2007.

Chapter Ten: Working Out and Chilling Out: Two Sides of the Same Chemopreventive Coin

Armaiz-Pena GN, Lutgendorf SK, Cole SW, et al., "Neuroendocrine modulation of cancer progression," *Brain Behav Immun* 23, no. 1 (January 2009): 10–5.

Carlson LE, Speca M, Faris P, et al., "One year pre-post intervention follow-up of psychological, immune, endocrine and blood pressure outcomes of mindfulness-based stress reduction (MBSR) in breast and prostate cancer outpatients," *Brain Behav Immun* 21, no. 8 (2007): 1038–49.

Frattaroli J, Weidner G, Dnistrian AM, et al., "Clinical events in the Prostate Cancer Lifestyle Trial: results from two years of follow-up," *Urology* 72, no. 6 (December 2008): 1319–23.

Kenfield SA, Stampfer MJ, Giovannucci E, "Physical activity and survival after prostate cancer diagnosis in the health professionals follow-up study," *J Clin Oncol* 29, no. 6 (February 2011): 726–32.

Moreno-Smith M, Lutgendorf SK, Sood AK, "Impact of stress on cancer metastasis," *Future Oncol* 6, no. 12 (December 2010): 1863–81.

Ornish D, Weidner G, Fair WR, et al., "Intensive lifestyle changes may affect the progression of prostate cancer," *J Urol* 174, no. 3 (September 2005): 1065–9.

Ornish D, Magbanua MJ, Weidner G, "Changes in prostate gene expression in men undergoing an intensive nutrition and lifestyle intervention," *Proc Natl Acad Sci USA* 105, no. 24 (June 2008): 8369–74.

Chapter 11: The "Growing Problem": Integrative Diagnosis and Treatment of Benign Prostatic Hyperplasia

Barton MK, "Few physicians prescribe 5-alpha reductase inhibitors for prostate cancer prevention," *CA Cancer J Clin* 61, no. 1 (January–February 2011): 1–2.

Chrubasik JE, Roufogalis BD, Wagner H, "A comprehensive review on stinging nettle effect and efficacy profiles. Part II: Urticae radix," *Phytomed* 14, no. 7 (August 2007): 568–79.

Greco KA, McVary KT, "The role of combination medical therapy in benign prostatic hyperplasia," *Int J Impot Res* 20 (December 2008): Suppl 3: S33–43.

Kristal AR, Arnold KB, Schenk JM, et al., "Dietary patterns, supplement use, and the risk of symptomatic benign prostatic hyperplasia: results from the prostate cancer prevention trial," *Am J Epidemiol* 167, no. 8 (2007): 925–34.

Schleich S, Papaioannou M, Baniahmad A, et al., "Extracts from Pygeum africanum and other ethnobotanical species with antiandrogenic activity," *Planta Med* 72, no. 9 (July 2006): 807–13.

Sinescu I, Geavlete P, Multescu R, et al., "Long-term efficacy of Serenoa repens treatment in patients with mild and moderate symptomatic benign prostatic hyperplasia," *Urol Int* (February 2011).

Quiles MT, Arbos MA, Fraga A, et al., "Antiproliferative and apoptotic effects of the herbal agent Pygeum africanum on cultured prostate stromal cells from patients with benign prostatic hyperplasia," *Prostate* 70, no. 10 (July 2010: 1044–53.

Wilt T, MacDonald R, Ishani A, "Cernilton for benign prostatic hyperplasia," *Cochrane Database Syst Rev* 2 (2000): CD001042.

Wilt T, Ishani A, MacDonald R, et al, "Beta-sitosterols for benign prostatic hyperplasia," *Cochrane Database System Reviews* 2 (2000): CD001043.

Xu J, Qian WQ, Song JD, "A comparative study on different doses of cernilton for preventing the clinical progression of benign prostatic hyperplasia," *Zhonghua Nan Ke Xue* 14, no. 6 (June 2008): 533–7.

Chapter 12: A Pain In the Prostate: Integrative Diagnosis and Therapy of Prostatitis

Anderson RU, Orenberg EK, Morey A, et al., "Stress-induced hypothalamus-pituitary-adrenal axis responses and disturbances in psychological profiles in men with chronic prostatitis/pelvic pain syndromes," *J Urol* 182, no. 5 (November 2009): 2319–2324.

Apolikhin OI, Aliaev IuG, Sivkov AV, et al, "A comparative clinical randomized trial of cernilton efficacy and safety in patients with chronic abacterial prostatitis," *Urologiia* 1 (January-February 2010): 29–34.

Capodice JL, Jin Z, Bemis DL, et al., "A pilot study on acupuncture for lower urinary tract symptoms related to chronic prostatitis/chronic pelvic pain," *Chin Med* 2 (2007): 1.

Wagenlehner FM, Schneider H, Ludwig M, et al, "A pollen extract (Cernilton) in patients with inflammatory chronic prostatitis-chronic pelvic pain syndrome: a multicentre, randomized, prospective, double-blind, placebo-controlled phase 3 study," *Eur Urol* 56, no. 3 (September 2009): 544–51.

Wise D, Anderson R, *A Headache in the Pelvis*, 6th ed. Occidental, CA: National Center for Pelvic Pain, 2010.

Yavascaoglu I, et al., "Role of ejaculate in the therapy of chronic non-bacterial prostatitis," *Int J Urol* 6 (1999): 130–4.

INDEX

Underscored page references indicate boxed text and charts.